Advances in Oto-Rhino-Laryngology

Vol. 81

Series Editor

Patrick J. Bradley Nottingham

Advances in Hearing Rehabilitation

Volume Editors

Simon K.W. Lloyd Manchester

Neil P. Donnelly Cambridge

46 figures, 23 in color, and 10 tables, 2018

KARGER

Basel · Freiburg · Paris · London · New York · Chennai · New Delhi ·
Bangkok · Beijing · Shanghai · Tokyo · Kuala Lumpur · Singapore · Sydney

Simon K.W. Lloyd
Honorary Clinical Professor of Otolaryngology and Consultant Otologist
University Department of Otolaryngology Head and Neck Surgery
Peter Mount House
Manchester Royal Infirmary
Manchester M13 9WL (UK)

Neil P. Donnelly
Consultant Otoneurological and Skull Base Surgeon
Department of Otolaryngology
Cambridge University Hospitals NHS Foundation Trust
Cambridge CB2 2QQ (UK)

Library of Congress Cataloging-in-Publication Data

Names: Lloyd, Simon (Simon Kingsley Wickham), editor. | Donnelly, Neil, 1972- editor.
Title: Advances in hearing rehabilitation / volume editors, Simon K.W. Lloyd, Neil Donnelly.
Other titles: Advances in oto-rhino-laryngology ; v. 81. 0065-3071
Description: Basel ; New York : Karger, 2018. | Series: Advances in oto-rhino-laryngology, ISSN 0065-3071 ; vol. 81 | Includes bibliographical references and indexes.
Identifiers: LCCN 2018004767| ISBN 9783318063141 (hard cover : alk. paper) | ISBN 9783318063158 (electronic version)
Subjects: | MESH: Cochlear Implantation | Correction of Hearing Impairment | Ear Diseases--rehabilitation | Ear, Middle--pathology
Classification: LCC RF300 | NLM WV 274 | DDC 617.8/9--dc23 LC record available at https://lccn.loc.gov/2018004767

Bibliographic Indices. This publication is listed in bibliographic services, including Current Contents® and Index Medicus.

www.karger.com
Printed on acid-free and non-aging paper (ISO 9706)
ISSN 0065–3071
e-ISSN 1662–2847
ISBN 978–3–318–06314–1
e-ISBN 978–3–318–06315–8

Contents

Preface

According to the World Health Organization, hearing loss ranks seventh as a cause for disease burden with 26 million years of healthy life lost globally each year. There is estimated to be 630 million people worldwide affected by some kind of hearing loss. On an individual level, the effect of hearing loss was eloquently summed up by Helen Keller, a remarkable American woman who lived around the turn of the 20th century and dedicated her life to social reform. She was rendered both blind and deaf at the age of 19 months following Scarlett fever and described blindness as separating people from things but deafness as separating people from people. Thus, hearing loss is an important cause of social isolation with both psychological and economic implications.

In the early 21st century, we are incredibly fortunate to be able to offer effective hearing rehabilitation to most patients with hearing loss, a situation unique among sensory losses. There has been a progressive improvement in hearing aid technologies, and surgical reconstruction of conductive hearing losses has become increasingly reliable with improvements in surgical technique and prosthesis design. The most dynamic area of development in the field of hearing rehabilitation is, however, implantation otology. Cochlear implants have been in mainstream clinical use for 30 years and have revolutionized the lives of those with acquired and congenital profound sensorineural hearing loss. Implantable hearing aids have proliferated over the past 15 years and now fill the gap between hearing aids and cochlear implants as well as offering an alternative means of rehabilitation for those that cannot wear traditional hearing aids. For those that do not have a functional cochlear nerve or have a cochlea that is absent or significantly deformed, auditory brainstem implantation now has a proven track record in offering limited access to hearing.

This book brings together some of the world's leading experts in hearing restoration to discuss recent advances in all aspects of hearing implantation otology. Chapters review the evidence behind the current applications of the wide range of hearing implants available for different types of hearing loss. The focus is on who should be implanted, with which device and how the outcomes can be optimized. There are contributions from authors leading in the extended applications of implantation otology and those horizon spotting for the next developments within this exciting field. New imaging techniques for the middle and inner ear are explored as well as innovations to improve Eustachian tube function.

We are very grateful to all the contributors for the enormous effort put into producing this book. It is aimed at otolaryngologists, audiologists and hearing rehabilitation professionals, and we very much hopeful that it will be a useful resource in providing a detailed overview of the current state-of-the-art in hearing rehabilitation.

Simon K.W. Lloyd, Manchester
Neil P. Donnelly, Cambridge

Lloyd SKW, Donnelly NP (eds): Advances in Hearing Rehabilitation.
Adv Otorhinolaryngol. Basel, Karger, 2018, vol 81, pp 1–13 (DOI: 10.1159/000485576)

New Imaging Modalities in Otology

Manohar Bance[a] · Andrzej Zarowski[b] · Robert A. Adamson[c] · Jan W. Casselman[d]

[a]Department of Otolaryngology, Addenbrookes Hospital, Cambridge, UK and University of Cambridge, Cambridge, UK;
[b]European Institute for Otolaryngology, Head and Neck Surgery, Sint Augustinus Hospital, Antwerp, Belgium;
[c]Department of Biomedical Engineering and Division of Otolaryngology, Dalhousie University, Halifax, NS, Canada;
[d]Department of Radiology, Medical Imaging, Sint Jan Hospital, Bruges, Belgium

Abstract

Despite steady improvements in cross-sectional imaging of the ear, current technologies still have limitations in terms of resolution, diagnosis, functional assessment and safety. In this chapter, state-of-the-art imaging techniques in current clinical practice are presented including cone-beam computerized tomography, non-echo planar imaging magnetic resonance imaging, imaging for labyrinthine hydrops and imaging of the central auditory pathways. Potential future imaging modalities are also presented, including optical coherence tomography (OCT) and high-frequency ultrasound (HFUS) of the ear. These experimental modalities offer new opportunities for the assessment of ear structure and function. For example, middle ear structures can be visualized through the tympanic membrane, basilar membrane vibrations can be assessed through the round window and the passage of cochlear implants can be assessed in decalcified cochlear. Functional assessment of the middle ear using Doppler techniques are also discussed, including measurement of tympanic membrane and middle ear vibration amplitudes, visualization of dynamic changes, such as tensor tympani movements and movement of the tympanic membrane with breathing. These new modalities currently have limitations that preclude mainstream clinical use. For example, OCT is limited by the optical scattering of the thickened tympanic membrane and HFUS needs a coupling medium such as gel or fluid from the transducer to the imaged structure although it can visualize through thicker tissues. Nevertheless, further development of these novel techniques may provide an enhanced ability to assess the ear in conjunction with current technologies.

Introduction

There are many anatomical and pathological aspects of the ear that are not well imaged by currently accessible technologies. While the resolutions of CT and MRI have improved steadily over time [1], these technologies still lack the resolution to clearly define middle ear or inner ear pathologies in sufficient detail to make precise clinical diagnoses or decisions, despite the impressive imaging available. Other drawbacks of current technologies are the exposure to ionizing radiation from CT imaging, and the artifacts and movement created in both CT and MRI from metallic or magnetic implants. Many structures in the middle and inner ears that are clinically important are in the millimeter and sub-millimeter ond-look surgery in the detection of recurrent or residual cholesteatoma, and can therefore save many patients unnecessary exploratory surgery. The major limitation of the technique is its inability to depict cholesteatoma smaller than 2 mm. It also lacks anatomical information and precise localization of cholesteatoma is not possible on these images. This can be solved by "matching" and "superposition" or "fusion" of the CT and MRI images (Fig. 3, 4).

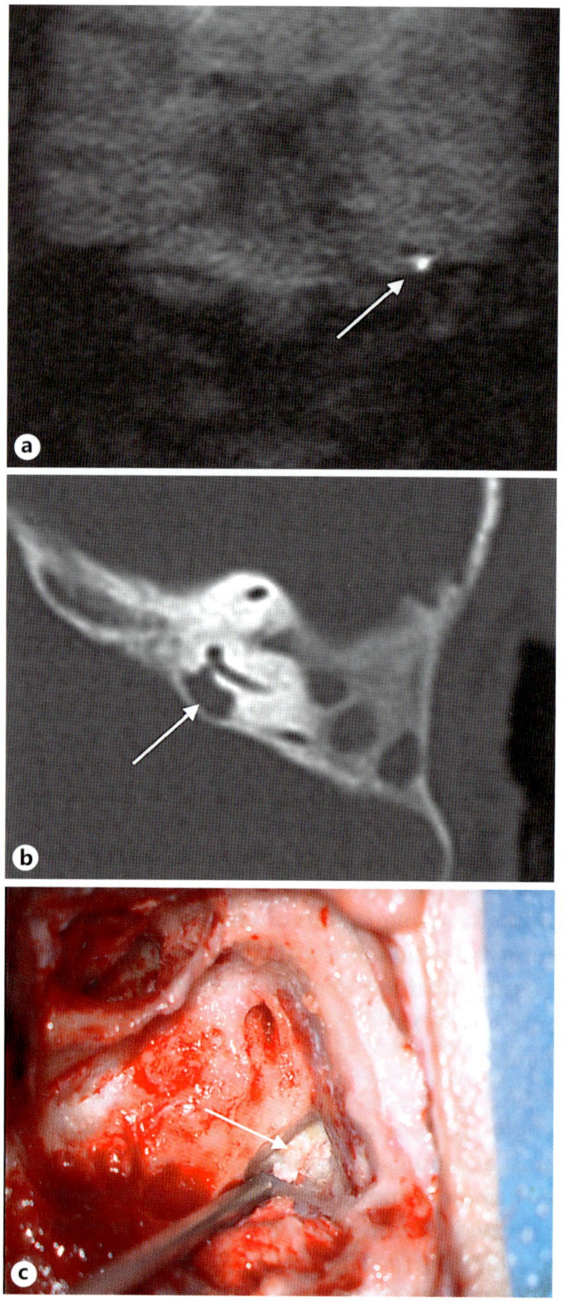

Fig. 3. Coronal B-1000 non-EPI DWI image (**a**), axial CBCT image (**b**), intraoperative view (**c**): White arrows show a small cholesteatoma in a small aerated and opacified cell in the petrous apex, located deep in the SCC. Without surgical-radiological correlation it would have been impossible to find this lesion.

MRI 3D FLAIR Hydrops Sequences

A new indication for MRI is the visualization of endolymphatic hydrops. It is performed after the injection of gadolinium contrast. Gadolinium administration can be intratympanic [3], intrathecal or intravenous. Intratympanic administration of gadolinium results in better image quality and higher contrast but it is invasive. Intravenous administration is less invasive and easier to perform, but requires a double dose and has poorer image quality.

This technique is based on the principle that gadolinium is able to pass through the normal "blood-perilymph" barrier but cannot pass through the "blood-endolymph" barrier, so that the perilymph will enhance and the endolymph will not. As result, the non-enhancing endolymphatic spaces (the saccule and the utricle) will be visualized on the background of the perilymph-filled vestibule. The normal scala media is too small to visualize, so the cochlea will show only enhancing scala tympani and scala vestibuli.

In hydropic ears, enlarged confluent non-enhancing endolymphatic areas inside the vestibule will be visible. If this area is still surrounded by an enhancing rim of perilymph, grade 1 vestibular hydrops may be diagnosed (Fig. 5). If the whole vestibular space is taken by the hydrops, we define it as grades 2 vestibular hydrops. In grade 1 cochlear hydrops, black spots are visible at the edges of the cochlea ("Christmas tree" image). In

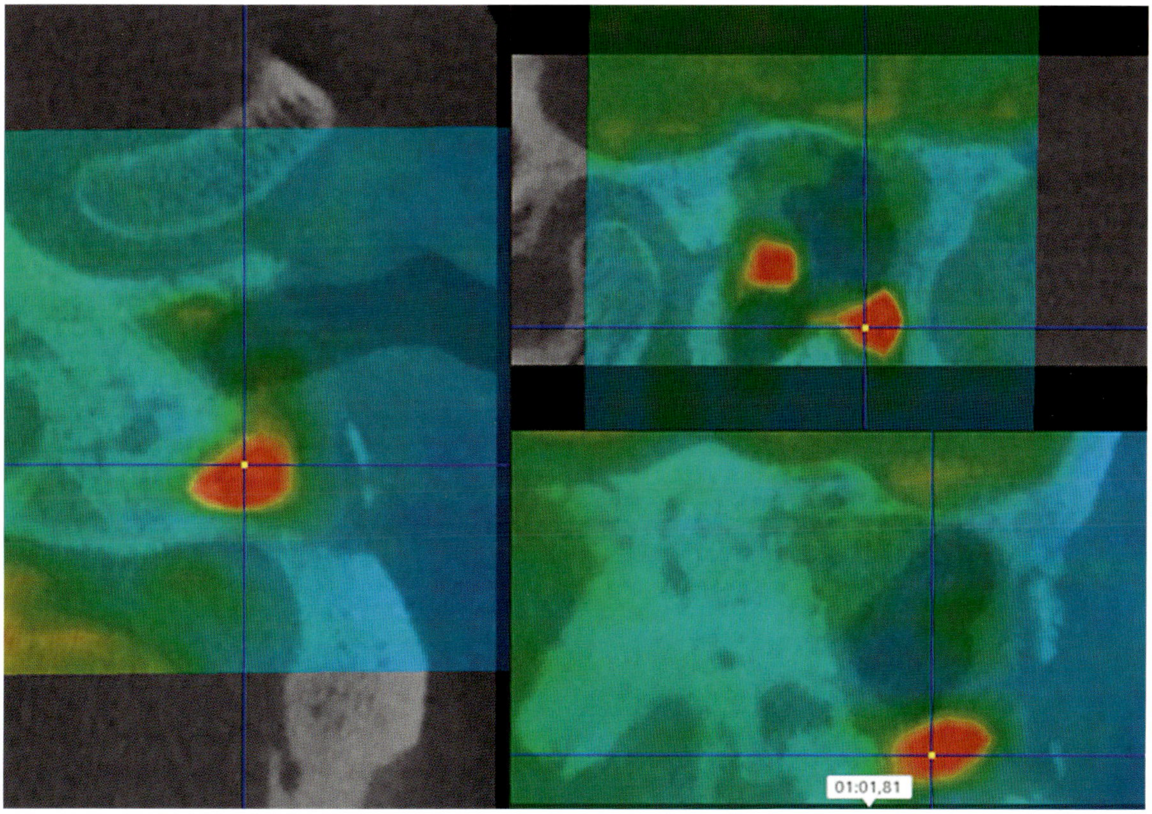

Fig. 4. Axial, sagittal and coronal CBCT and MRI non-EPI DWI "fusion" images: Postoperative evaluation showing 2 recidive/residual cholesteatomas visualized in axial, sagittal and coronal planes by "matching" and "superposition" or "fusion" of a 3T non-EPI DWI image and a CBCT image obtained using dedicated workstations and software.

grade 2 cochlear hydrops, black horizontal strips are observed in the cochlea and represent the non-enhancing hydropic scala media which completely replaces the enhancing perilymph in the scala vestibuli, even in the area around the modiolus.

The maximum enhancement of perilymph is seen 4 h after intravenous gadolinium administration. Therefore, MR imaging must be performed 4 h after the injection. Since enhancement is weak after intravenous administration of the contrast, a double dose of gadolinium is needed and the more sensitive FLAIR sequence is used. To improve the spatial resolution, 3D-FLAIR is applied. Obtaining high resolution requires sequences of 10–15 min so good immobilization of the head is necessary, for example, fixation with the use of. To optimize the signal-to-noise ratio (SNR), a 32-channel coil is used and when possible the coil elements closest to the ears are even positioned between the auricles and the headphones to further increase SNR.

Clinical Utility

Meniere's disease is traditionally diagnosed using clinical indicators according to the criteria of the American Academy of Otolaryngology – Head and Neck Surgery of 1995 and the new criteria of the Barany Society 2016 [4, 5]. However, these anamnestic-based diagnostic criteria are

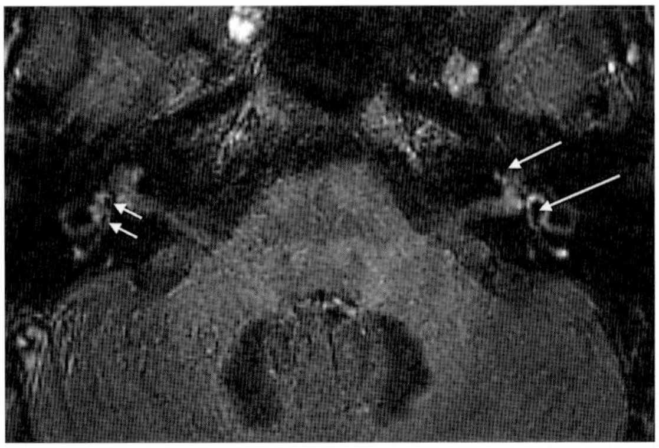

Fig. 5. Endolymphatic hydrops on the left side visualized on a contrast-enhanced 3D-FLAIR image: Long white arrow points to confluent signal-void area in the left vestibulum (hydrops grade 1). Shorter white arrow points to hydropic scala media in the left cochlea (hydrops grade 1). Right ear is normal. Very short white arrowheads show normal anatomy of the sacculus and utriculus on the right side.

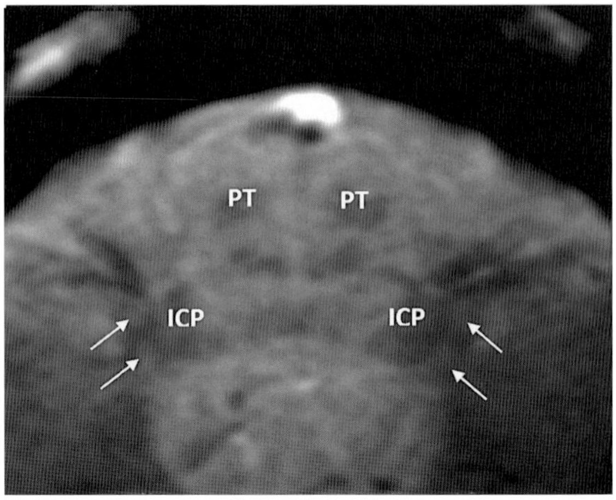

Fig. 6. Visualization of the cochlear nuclei on an axial m-FFE image: Short white arrows show bilaterally normal ventral and dorsal cochlear nuclei visible as light grey structures on the dark grey background of the myelinated inferior cerebellar pedunculus (ICP). Dark myelinated pyramidal tracts (PT) are also visible in the brainstem.

intrinsically imprecise and cause diagnostic false positive and negative results. This has traditionally made objective assessment of treatment modalities almost impossible [6]. MRI hydrops imaging is able to identify patients with definite hydrops with a sensitivity and specificity of more than 90% and may be helpful in the reassessment of the efficacy of treatments with a traditionally poor evidence base, for example, sac surgery.

MRI Multi-Echo Fast Field Echo Sequences

The Multi-Echo Fast Field Echo (mFFE) sequence is very useful for the visualization of the brainstem nuclei (Fig. 6). The unmyelinated fibers and nuclei appear as grey structures on the background of the black myelinated fibers.

Clinical Utility

Bilateral congenital deafness can currently be successfully treated by cochlear implantation. This option is, however, not available for children born with bilateral aplasia of the cochlear nerve. For such children, the only remaining functional option is brainstem implantation. The auditory outcomes of brainstem implantation in children with no cochlear nerves are very variable, ranging from no audition to open-set speech discrimination [7, 8]. The reasons for this huge variability in obtained results are not very well understood. One of the potential explanations could be concomitant under-development of aberrantly located cochlear nuclei away from the lateral recess of the 4th ventricle where the brainstem implant electrode is being placed.

Application of the mFFE sequence for the visualization of the cochlear nuclei does, however, have its limitations which are related to the age of the child. Myelinization of the brainstem structures surrounding the cochlear nuclei has to be sufficient to enable visualization of these auditory nuclei. This is usually only the case at the age of 2 years.

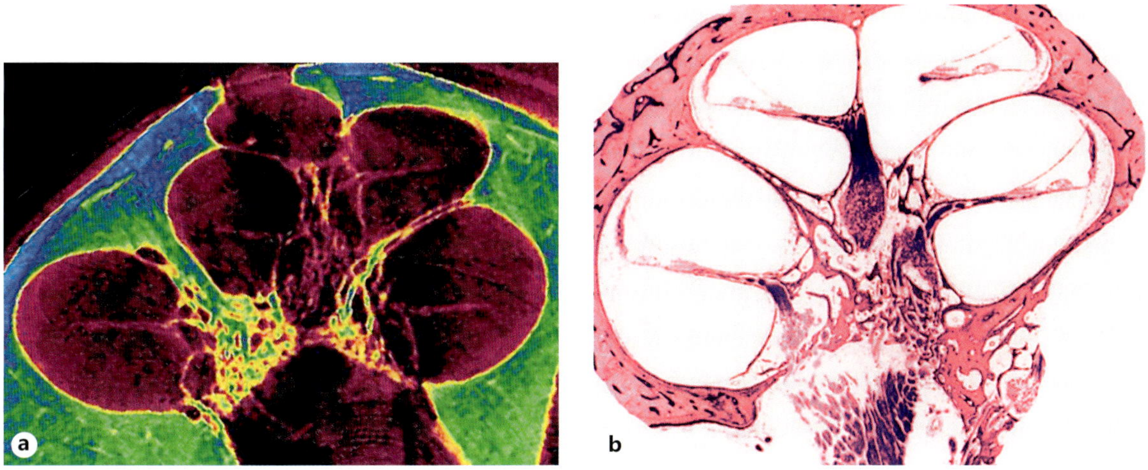

Fig. 7. X-ray micro-CT (**a**), histological image of the human cochlea (**b**): (**a**) shows an X-ray micro-CT investigation (Skyscan-1076 scanner) of the cochlea with 18 micron pixel size and Ti-filter. On (**b**), corresponding histological section of the human cochlea is shown.

X-Ray Microtomography

Another potentially interesting experimental imaging technique that helps in the visualization of the middle and inner ears is X-ray microtomography (micro-CT).

The concept of micro-CT is similar to clinical CT with an X-ray source and detector rotating around the region of interest. However, unlike classical CT scanners that have linear detectors scanning one layer after another, micro-CT uses 2 CCD cameras as a 2D detector providing cross-section up to 4,000 × 4,000 pixels. The 2D detector reduces the scanning time dramatically compared to linear detectors. Isotropic datasets that allow visualization of any arbitrary cross-section in any orientation may be obtained. Micro-CT machines have a reduced field of view (up to 68 mm in diameter and 200 mm long) but this is compensated by very high resolution (down to 9 micron). This high resolution is not related to the object size.

Micro-CT is a powerful technique that allows visualization of the internal structure of opaque preparations [9, 10]. In biomedical research, micro-CT has not only been applied for studying bones and calcified tissues [11–14], but also for imaging soft tissues such as lung tumors [15]. One of the potential new applications of micro-CT is the visualization of the inner ear tissues with semi-histological quality (Fig. 7) and evaluation of the surgical aspects of newly developed cochlear implant electrodes [16] (Fig. 8). Unfortunately, high radiation doses make it unsuitable for clinical practice, but it is a useful research tool that provides high resolution without the need for bone decalcification or extensive processing of the samples.

High-Frequency Ultrasound

Ultrasound imaging is a low-cost, real-time modality used widely throughout many areas of medicine. Conventional ultrasound technology operates by sending an acoustic stimulus at a frequency between 1 and 10 MHz into tissue and forming images from the reflections from tissue structures. High-frequency ultrasound (HFUS) operates in the same way, but at frequencies in the

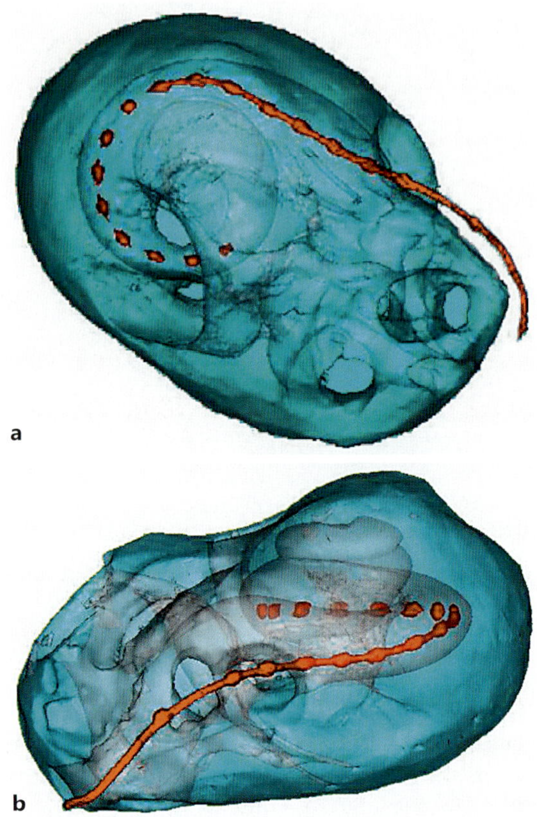

Fig. 8. 3-D reconstructions of the micro-CT images: Semi-transparent 3-D models of human cochlea with inserted cochlear implant electrode (Advanced Bionics Hi-Focus II electrode with 16 contacts). Side view (**a**). View from above (**b**).

20–100 MHz range. The higher frequency allows for improved axial and lateral resolutions of the order of 10's of microns compared to 100's of microns for conventional ultrasound, but at the expense of lower penetration in soft tissues (i.e., 10–15 mm at 50 MHz) due to increased absorption and scattering [17–21]. HFUS is a promising technology for use in the auditory system where it can provide better resolution than MRI or CT of middle ear and inner ear structures [18, 20, 21]. It also offers the potential of being able to measure the vibration of structures in both the middle and inner ears [18, 20], which could be an important new source of diagnostic information. Imaging requires a fluid acoustic coupling such as gel or liquid and this requires that the middle ear is filled with saline (unless there is already serous fluid present). Ultrasound imaging of the cochlea is possible through the round window with a drop of fluid or gel providing coupling [18]. Ultrasound is minimally attenuated by soft tissues, such as the tympanic membrane, round window folds or cholesteatoma or by middle ear effusion. While the need for direct acoustic coupling makes high-frequency ultrasound (HIFUS) imaging more invasive than some other modalities, it may have some application for specific disorders of the middle ear and offers great promise for intracochlear imaging.

Clinical Utility

The potential utility and resolution of HiFUS has been demonstrated in a cadaveric study undertaken by the authors using a 50 MHz annular array [17], demonstrating detailed resolution of individual ossicles and the basilar membrane through the round window. Vibrations of the basilar membrane in human cadaveric temporal bones in the region overlying the round window have subsequently been measured, using a 45 MHz pulsed-wave needle mounted single element probe [3]. Imaging of normal and pathological ear structures, through the eardrum, in a saline filled middle ear has also been demonstrated using a linear 50 MHz array (Fig. 9) [19–21]. Dynamic movement of the middle ear structures, in response to indentation of the eardrum and acoustic stimuli, was also easily measured although the coupling fluid does influence these measurements to some degree.

The cochlea is difficult to access through the otic capsule, because of the inability of ultrasound to penetrate bone but by decalcifying human temporal bones, it is possible to see areas outside the field of view afforded by the round window, and visualize a large portion of the basilar membrane. Figure 10 shows a decalcified cochlea with a co-

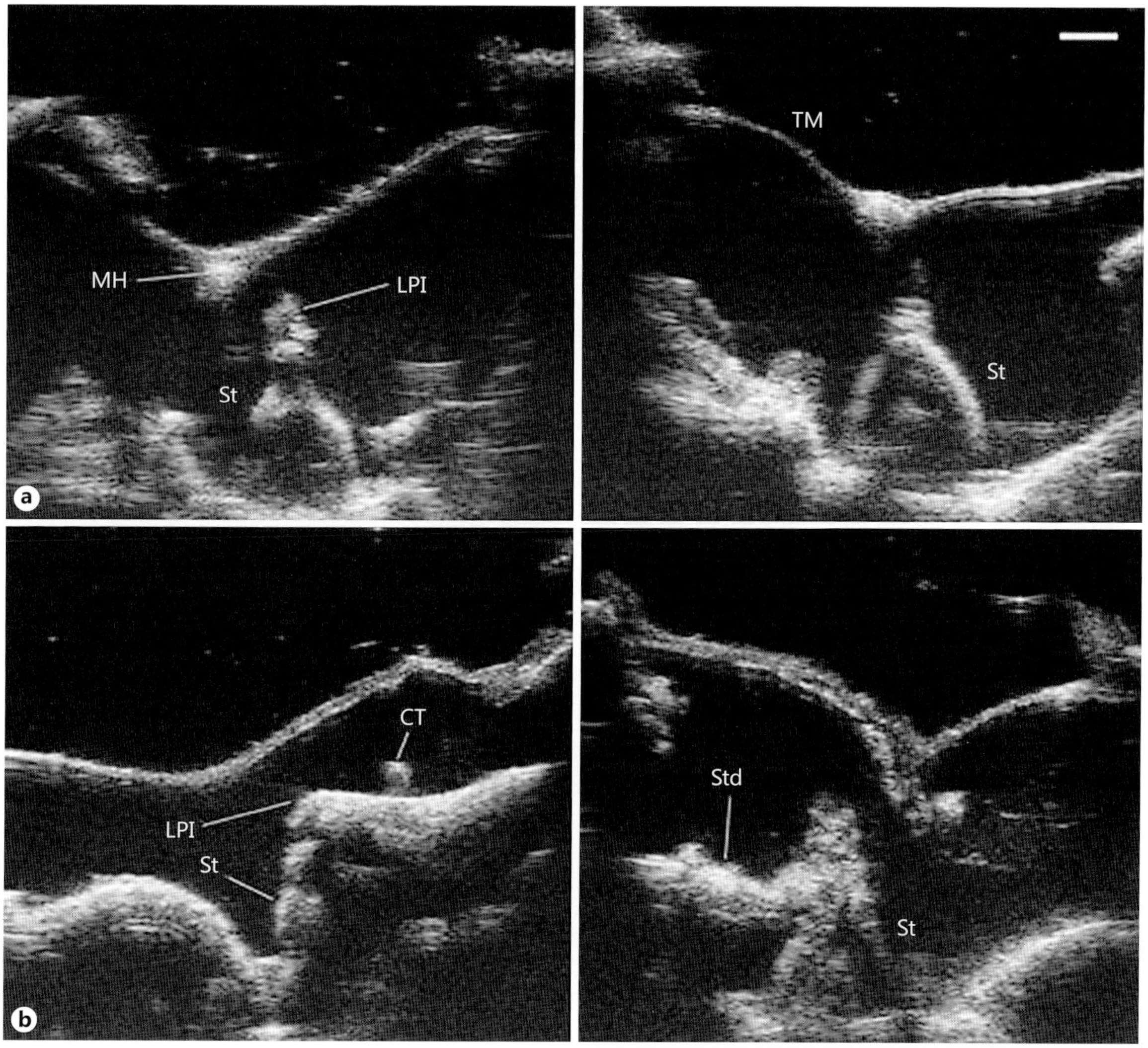

Fig. 9. a, **b** HFUS images of normal middle ears collected using a commercially available HFUS unit (Vevo 2100; VIsual-Sonics, Canada). Many structures are apparent, including the tympanic membrane (TM), malleus handle (MH), long process of the incus (LPI) and stapes (St). It is important to note that the imaging probe used for collecting these images could not be used clinically, as the ear canal must be totally removed due to the probe size and limited viewing depth of 10 mm (Fig. 1c, d). Good continuity contact between the tympanic membrane (TM), a cartilage interposer, and the head of a total ossicular replacement prosthesis (TORP) was observed (top-left panel), as was good contact between a partial ossicular replacement prosthesis (PORP) and the head of the stapes (St; top-right panel). Scale bar = 1 mm.

chlear implant inside it. This could be a powerful tool for understanding how implants interact with the structures inside the cochlea, as the imaging is dynamic, and the path of the electrode array can be followed.

Because linear arrays are too large to fit through the ear canal, a 64-element phased array that can fit into the ear canal is currently under development, and may even be able to look into the cochlea through the round window [22].

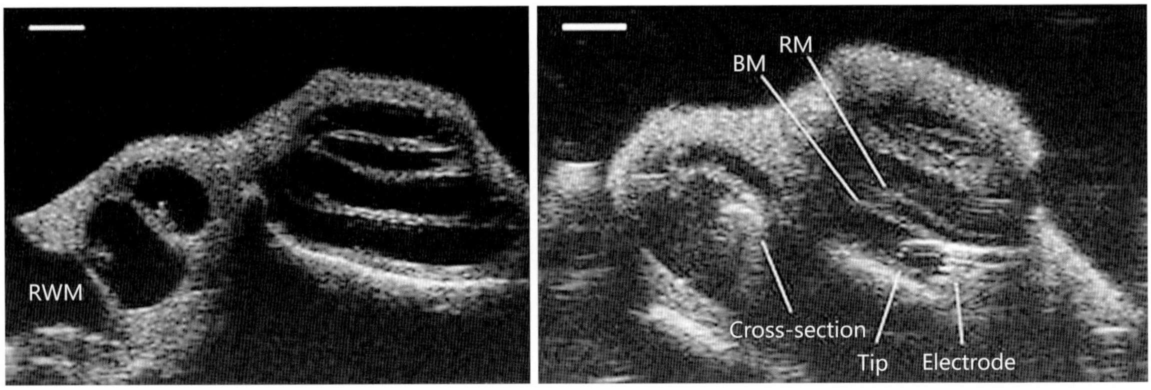

Fig. 10. HFUS images of a decalcified human cochlea with a modiolar image section plane, collected using the VisualSonics imaging system. The right panel shows the same cochlea implanted with a Cochlear slim straight array (implant aspects labelled with italics). RWM, round window membrane; BM, basilar membrane; RM, Reissner's membrane. Scale bars = 1 mm.

Optical Coherence Tomography

Optical Coherence Tomography (OCT) is an emerging interferometric optical imaging technology that provides depth-resolved images of the optical reflectivity of tissue structures [23]. OCT works by splitting light into a reference and sample arm. The sample arm light is directed at the tissue to be imaged, while the reference arm light is reflected back and interfered with light reflecting from the tissue. With a broadband light source, depth-resolved image lines can be obtained along the sample beam either by changing the length of the reference arm in time-domain OCT [24, 25] or by fixing the reference arm length and recording the spectrum of the interfered light in spectral-domain OCT [26]. Alternatively, a narrow-band laser source capable of being swept in time may be used as the source in swept-source OCT [27], in which case the image line can be obtained from the time course of the interferogram.

OCT was first proposed for use in ear imaging by Pitris et al. [24], and, as the technology has advanced, interest has grown in its use as a clinical tool, particularly for imaging of the tympanic membrane [28, 29]. Recently, researchers have explored the potential of OCT for imaging the middle ear through the tympanic membrane as well [25, 26]. OCT is undertaken down the ear canal and can be configured to provide Doppler information about the vibration of ear structures in response to sound. Doppler information has been shown to be useful for diagnosing disorders that are not apparent in purely anatomical OCT images [26].

Clinical Utility

Because the TM is translucent, OCT allows imaging of the middle ear structures through the TM. Unlike HFUS, no contact or coupling medium is required between the light source and imaged structures making OCT a non-invasive, non-contact modality. In the past, OCT has been used in vivo to measure tympanic membrane thickness, and infer the presence of biofilm and middle ear infection [26], but with little anatomical resolution. While these techniques were not able to image the entire middle ear volume due to limited depth range, real-time imaging of the entire middle ear volume in vivo using swept-source OCT in both 2D and 3D has recently been demonstrated by the authors (Fig. 11). OCT images such as this one could potentially be used to look in detail at disorders of the TM, such as granular myringitis, and thickening and blunting of the TM. OCT can

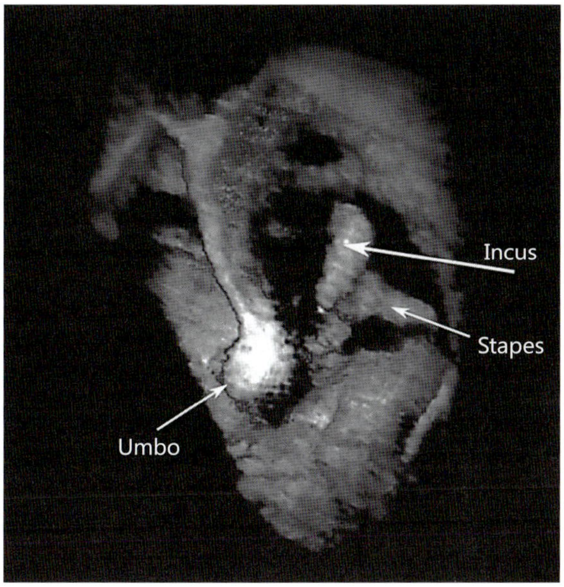

Fig. 11. OCT image of cadaveric middle ear through the TM, showing visualization of the incus, the stapes and the umbo.

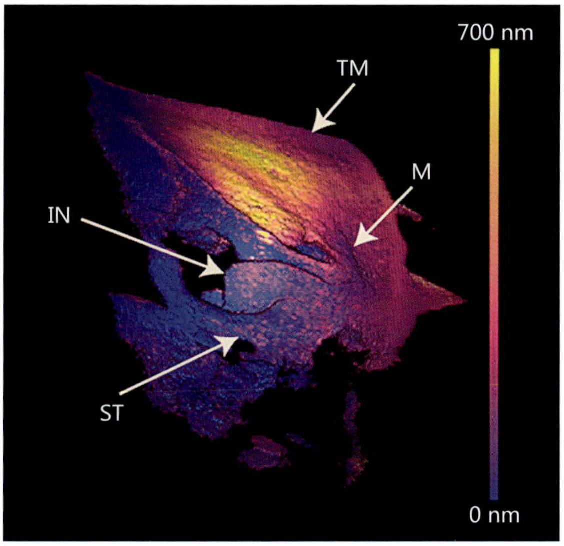

Fig. 12. OCT "Vibrogram" of the middle ear, showing vibration amplitude of middle ear structures measured with a 3D volumetric acquisition through the TM. Redder hues are higher amplitudes, and bluer hues are lower amplitudes of vibration. TM, tympanic membrane; IN, Incus; ST, stapes; M, malleus. Stimulation frequency is 500 Hz.

also measure the vibration of structures in the middle ear, and perform a "vibrogram" [30] (Fig. 12). Doppler OCT imaging has the capacity to revolutionize our understanding of why some middle ears have conductive hearing loss, why some prostheses work and others do not, and what the effects of healing are on vibration responses of the ear.

Limitations of OCT and HFUS

Most ears with pathology show anatomical abnormalities that can limit the use of OCT or HFUS. While pathologies such as otosclerosis present with relatively normal TMs, and can be imaged with OCT, other pathologies and surgical interventions such as cartilage tympanoplasty, often thicken the eardrum, impeding light penetration and making OCT imaging impossible. In such cases, HFUS offers a promising alternative owing to its superior soft-tissue penetration. HFUS, however, requires that the middle ear either have saline, serous effusion, or tissue (e.g., granulation) in it.

A common limitation to both OCT and HFUS is their inability to image through bone. Pathologies of interest, such as cholesteatoma, are often hidden in the epitympanum by bone and so cannot be visualized easily with these modalities as currently implemented. However, it may be possible to build side-looking probes that might be able to look at these areas.

Conclusion

Current imaging techniques provide excellent anatomical information but have limitations in resolution and do not provide functional information. There are several new imaging modalities that show promise either as research tools or in clinical practice to address these limitations and some of these may enter the mainstream use in the coming years.

Acknowledgments

The following also made a significant contribution to this chapter: De Foer B, Offeciers FE, Somers T, van Dinther J, Landry TG, McDougall D, Brown J, Farrell J, Rainsbury JW. Dr. Jeremy Brown (Assoc. Prof. Biomedical Engineering Dalhousie University, Canada) was responsible for the high frequency ultrasound work. Dr. Tom Landry and Dr. James Rainsbury (EAR lab, Dalhousie University, Canada) performed the cadaveric imaging.

References

1 Juliano AF, Ginat DT, Moonis G: Imaging review of the temporal bone: part I. Anatomy and inflammatory and neoplastic processes. Radiology 2013;269:17–33.
2 Lagleyre S, Sorrentino T, Calmels MN, et al: Reliability of high-resolution CT scan in diagnosis of otosclerosis. Otol and Neurotol 2009;30:1152–1159.
3 Nakashima T, Naganawa S, Sugiura M, Teranishi M, Sone M, Hayashi H, Nakata S, Katayama N, Ishida IM: Visualization of endolymphatic hydrops in patients with Meniere's disease. Laryngoscope 2007;117:415–420.
4 Committee on Hearing and Equilibrium guidelines for the diagnosis and evaluation of therapy in Menière's disease. American Academy of Otolaryngology-Head and Neck Foundation, Inc. Otolaryngol Head Neck Surg 1995;113:181–185.
5 Lopez-Escamez JA, Carey J, Chung WH, Goebel JA, Magnusson M, Mandalà M, Newman-Toker DE, Strupp M, Suzuki M, Trabalzini F, Bisdorff A: Diagnostic criteria for Menière's disease. Consensus document of the Bárány Society, the Japan Society for Equilibrium Research, the European Academy of Otology and Neurotology (EAONO), the American Academy of Otolaryngology-Head and Neck Surgery (AAO-HNS) and the Korean Balance Society. Acta Otorrinolaringol Esp 2016;67:1–7.
6 Thomsen J, Bretlau P, Tos M, Johnsen NJ: Ménière's disease: endolymphatic sac decompression compared with sham (placebo) decompression. Ann N Y Acad Sci 1981;374:820–830.
7 Sennaroglu L, Colletti V, Manrique M, Laszig R, Offeciers E, Saeed S, Ramsden R, Sarac S, Freeman S, Andersen HR, Zarowski A, Ziyal I, Sollmann WP, Kaminsky J, Bejarano B, Atas A, Sennaroglu G, Yucel E, Sevinc S, Colletti L, Huarte A, Henderson L, Wesarg T, Konradsson K: Auditory brainstem implantation in children and non-neurofibromatosis type 2 patients: a consensus statement. Otol Neurotol 2011;32:187–191.
8 Sennaroğlu L, Sennaroğlu G, Yücel E, Bilginer B, Atay G, Bajin MD, Mocan BÖ, Yaral M, Aslan F, Çnar BÇ, Özkan B, Batuk MÖ, Kirazl ÇE, Karakaya J, Ataş A, Saraç S, Ziyal İ: Long-term results of ABI in children with severe inner ear malformations. Otol Neurotol 2016;37:865–872.
9 Sasov A, Van Dyck D: Desktop x-ray microscopy and microtomography. J Microsc 1998;191:151–158.
10 Boyde A, De Clerck NM, Sasov A: MicroCT of Bones and Soft Tissues. Microsc Anal (UK Ed) 2000;76:70.
11 De Clerck NM, Van Dyck D, Postnov AA: Non-invasive high-resolution µCT of the inner structure of living snimals. Microsc Anal 2003;81:13–15.
12 Postnov A, De Clerck N, Sasov A, Van Dyck D: 3D in-vivo X-ray microtomography of living snails. J Microsc 2002;205:201–205.
13 Postnov AA, Vinogradov AV, Van Dyck D, Saveliev SV, De Clerck NM: Quantitative analysis of bone mineral content by x-ray microtomography. Physiol Meas 2003;24:165–178.
14 Waarsing JH, Day JS, van der Linden JC, Ederveen AG, Spanjers C, De Clerck N, Sasov A, Verhaar JA, Weinans H: Detecting and tracking local changes in the tibiae of individual rats: a novel method to analyse longitudinal in vivo micro-CT data. Bone 2004;34:163–169.
15 De Clerck NM, Meurrens K, Weiler H, Van Dyck D, Vanhoutte G, Terpstra P, Postnov AA: High resolution X-ray microtomography for the detection of lung tumors in living mice. Neoplasia 2004;6:374–379.
16 Postnov A, Zarowski A, De Clerck N, Vanpoucke F, Offeciers FE, Van Dyck D, Peeters S: High resolution micro-CT scanning as an innovative tool for evaluation of the surgical positioning of cochlear implant electrodes. Acta Otolaryngol 2006;126:467–474.
17 Brown JA, et al: High-frequency ex vivo ultrasound imaging of the auditory system. Ultrasound Med Biol 2009;35:1899–1907.
18 Torbatian Z, et al: Listening to the cochlea with high-frequency ultrasound. Ultrasound Med Biol 2012;38:2208–2217.
19 Foster FS, et al: A new 15–50 MHz array-based micro-ultrasound scanner for preclinical imaging. Ultrasound Med Biol 2009;35:1700–1708.
20 Landry TG, et al: Real-time imaging of in-vitro human middle ear using high frequency ultrasound. Hear Res 2015;326:1–7.
21 Rainsbury JW, et al: High frequency ex vivo ultrasound imaging of the middle ear to show simulated ossicular pathology. Otol Neurotol 2016;37:586–592.
22 Bezanson A, Adamson R, Brown J: Fabrication and performance of a miniaturized 64-element high-frequency endoscopic phased array. IEEE Trans Ultrason Ferroelectr Freq Control 2014;61:33–43.
23 Brezinski ME: Optical coherence tomography: principles and applications. Amsterdam/Boston, Academic Press, 2006.

24 Pitris C, Saunders KT, Fujimoto JG, Brezinski ME: High-resolution imaging of the middle ear with optical coherence tomography: a feasibility study. Arch Otolaryngol Head Neck Surg 2001;127:637–642.
25 MacDougall D, Rainsbury J, Brown J, Bance M, Adamson R: Optical coherence tomography system requirements for clinical diagnostic middle ear imaging. J Biomed Opt 2015;20:056008.
26 Subhash HM, Nguyen-Huynh A, Wang RK, Jacques SL, Choudhury N, Nuttall AL: Feasibility of spectral-domain phase-sensitive optical coherence tomography for middle ear vibrometry. J Biomed Opt 2012;17:060505.
27 Park J, Carbajal EF, Chen X, Oghalai JS, Applegate BE: Phase-sensitive optical coherence tomography using an Vernier-tuned distributed Bragg reflector swept laser in the mouse middle ear. Opt Lett 2014;39:6233–6236.
28 Djalilian HR, Ridgway J, Tam M, Sepehr A, Chen Z, Wong BJ: Imaging the human tympanic membrane using optical coherence tomography In vivo. Otol Neurotol 2008;29:1091–1094.
29 Monroy GL, Shelton RL, Nolan RM, Nguyen CT, Novak MA, Hill MC, McCormick DT, Boppart SA: Noninvasive depth-resolved optical measurements of the tympanic membrane and middle ear for differentiating otitis media: differentiation of Otitis Media Using OCT. Laryngoscope 2015;125:E276–E282.
30 Chang EW, Kobler JB, Yun SH: Subnanometer optical coherence tomographic vibrography. Opt Lett 2012;37:3678.

Prof. Manohar Bance
ENT Department of Otolaryngology, Addenbrookes Hospital
Hills Road, Box 48
Cambridge CB2 0QQ (UK)
E-Mail mlb59@cam.ac.uk

Dr. Andrzej Zarowski
European Institute for Otorhinolaryngology, Head and Neck Surgery, AZ Sint Augustinus
Oosterveldlaan 24
BE–2610 Wilrijk (Belgium)
E-Mail andrzej.zarowski@gza.be

Table 1. Classification of middle ear hearing reconstruction techniques

(A) Pressure gain at OW (PGOW) reconstruction

(I) Direct connection TM to residual ossicles

a Direct connection incus onto TM: (D-IOT- Wullstein type 2)

b **Direct connection stapes head onto TM: (D-SHOT-Wullstein type 3)**

(II) Connectors between TM and residual ossicles

Connecting	*Acronym*	*Current terminology or examples*
Stapes head onto TM	**SHOT**	**PORP**
Stapes head onto malleus	**SHOM**	**PORP**
Stapes head onto incus	SHOI	e.g. Cement, Applebaum
Stapes head onto both TM and malleus	SHOTM	PORP
Stapes head to artificial or relocated malleus	SHOAM	PORP to relocated malleus
Stapes footplate onto TM	**FOT**	**TORP**
Stapes footplate onto malleus	**FOM**	**TORP**
Stapes footplate onto incus	FOI	e.g. stapes piston on mobile footplate
Stapes footplate onto both TM and malleus	FOTM	
Stapes footplate onto relocated or artificial malleus	FOAM	e.g. TORP to relocated malleus
Vestibule to TM	VOT	TORP with stapedotomy
Vestibule to malleus	VOM	Malleostapediopexy
Vestibule to incus	**VOI**	**Standard stapedotomy**
Vestibule to both TM and malleus	VOB	
Vestibule to artificial or relocated malleus	VOAM	Rarely used
Incus to TM	IOM	Rarely used
Incus to malleus	IOT	e.g. cementing IM joint, rarely used

(B) OW access with RW protection (RoWPOWA) hearing reconstruction

RoWPOWA-FP: stapes footplate access (Wullstein type 4)

RoWPOWA-V: inner ear access with removal of stapes footplate (Wullstein type 5b)

RoWPOWA-HC: inner ear access with lateral canal fenestration (Wullstein type 5a)

In general, the lateral and medial and mid prosthesis interface/stabilizers should be specified, e.g. medial +/– footplate shoe, lateral +/– cartilage overlay, mid-shaft +/– cartilage or other stabilizer. The most commonly used are in bold face. PORP, partial ossicular replacement prosthesis; TORP, total ossicular replacement prosthesis.

3. It must transmit force efficiently, that is, not itself have high mechanical impedance, and be relatively rigid.

4. It should ideally be able to adapt to static pressure changes in the middle ear and maintain its efficiency.

5. It should be easy to place, with good surgical handling characteristics.

6. It should be easy to revise.

7. It should be stable in that it stays in position in the long and short term.

8. It should be relatively cheap and adaptable.

9. It should be compatible with imaging, for example, MRI or CT imaging, and not cause too much artefact.

It would be perhaps even better than the unreconstructed ear if it could reverse middle ear pathology by biological coatings that inhibit or reverse inflammatory processes.

Biocompatibility

The most biocompatible material will be autologous ossicle, for example, sculpted incus, but this is not necessarily the best fit or most easily available in many ears. Many allograft materials have been tried, particularly ceramics (e.g., hydroxyapatite, bioglass, aluminum oxide, ceravital), metals (e.g., titanium, platinum, gold, steel) and plastics (e.g., teflon, polyethylene).

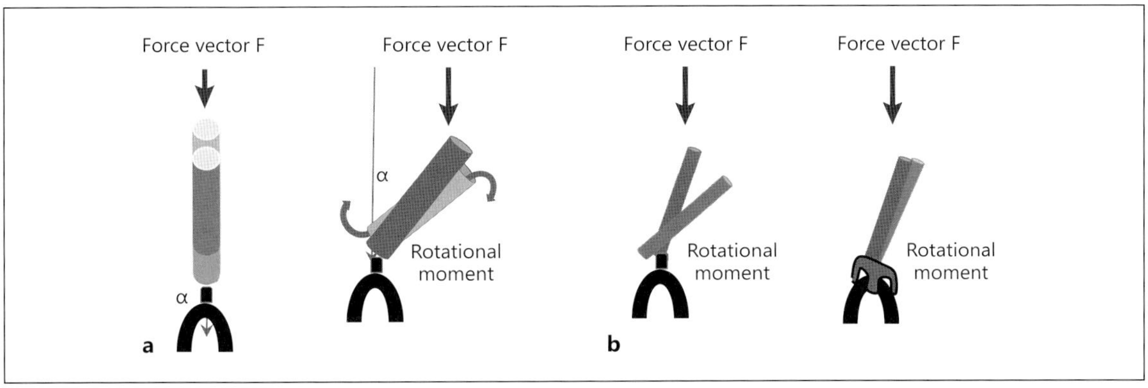

Fig. 1. a An in line-force vector is more likely to cause more translational movement, and less rotational movement than an eccentric force vector, which creates a rotational movement (**b**). By constraining the rotational movement with a cup-like arrangement, the rotational movement is constrained.

Biomaterials are commonly divided into bioinert, biotolerant or bioactive materials. Bioinert materials such as gold do not react with host tissues, but can still be extruded [8]. Biotolerant materials develop a coating which conceals them from the body. Examples are polyethylene (such as Plastipore®), but very high extrusion rates [9] have led to their disuse. The main advantage of these materials is that they can be easily shaped. Composites, such as Flex H/A(R) (hydroxyapatite and silastic) or HAPEX® (hydroxyapatite and polyethylene), retain some ability to be easily modified with substantially decreased excursion rates [10].

Bioactive materials, such as glass ceramics or hydroxyapatite, actually do cause some reaction by definition, and can be biodegraded, but the effect of this depends on the thickness of the material. Hydroxyapatite has stood the test of time. The most commonly used materials in modern middle ear prostheses are titanium metals and hydroxyapatites. Titanium implants are mostly bioinert, and seem to be well tolerated, with reported extrusion rates of 5% or less, even without cartilage interposition [11]. Most of the earlier materials such as Plastipore required cartilage cover to prevent extrusion.

Efficient Transfer of Force Vectors

One of the key areas where prostheses may fail in transmitting vibrations is by attenuating power across the coupling interfaces, primarily the interface from the TM to the prosthesis, and prosthesis and the remaining structures (typically stapes head (stapes head onto malleus [SHOM] or stapes head onto TM [SHOT]; Table 1), or the footplate (footplate onto malleus [FOM] or footplate onto TM [FOT]). There are 2 ways these losses can occur. The first is that there is a gap or compliance such as soft tissue across the interface, which does not transmit certain frequencies well. For instance, large compliances tend to absorb higher frequencies, which are lower amplitude vibrations. In the worst case, a gap will effectively not transmit any vibration energy. Another type of coupling losses at the interface arises if the piston-like in-line force vectors required to drive the stapes footplate efficiently are replaced with rotational movements, because the force vectors have a large rotational moment. Figure 1 show this schematically. The in-line force vector is actually the $\cos^2 \alpha$ of the angle in Figure 1, and much of the motion of an angulated prosthesis can be a rotational movement.

By constraining the rotational moment, it is possible to maximize the in-line piston like movement. This is much easier for a reconstruction to the stapes head than to the footplate (i.e., the SHOM and SHOT versus the FOM and FOT reconstructions in Table 1) and is likely one of the reasons that reconstructions utilizing the stapes head perform better than the stapes footplate [12]. Prosthetic designs that use a deep cup that limits the rotational movement will have a mechanical advantage in addition to a stability advantage. The cup should not be so deep that it contacts the promontory, it should not require excessive force to attach, nor result in necrosis of the superstructure and should be easy to revise.

On the footplate, this containment of the rotational movement is much harder to achieve, although people have described various methods to try and stabilize the medial end of the prosthesis including footplate shoes. Whilst they make sense mechanically, they also add damping and additional mechanical impedance, and the shoe can rotate on the footplate. In practice, these shoes can make it difficult to see that the footplate is contacted adequately and may be difficult to place. The ideal prosthesis would bond to the footplate, but this would make revisions difficult. In fact, the truly ideal prosthesis would bypass the footplate, and the impedance of the annular ligament, and transmit energy directly to the vestibular fluids. However, this presents a problem in chronic ear surgery as the ear might be infected or prone to future infections and the TM might medialize and push the prosthesis into the vestibule. In addition, the stapes footplate is mobile and perforating it risks pushing it into the vestibule. These considerations have militated against the use of direct to vestibule prostheses, despite their advantages.

Mechanical Properties of the Implant

The mechanical properties of the implant probably only have a minor effect on the transmission of vibrations, provided they meet some minimum criteria outlined below.

Rigidity: The implant has to be more rigid than the structures it is driving, otherwise the forces exerted on it will lead to bending and losses in its compliance rather than in delivering the force to the target. Compliances are likely to particularly affect the higher frequencies. In practice, almost all commercially available and autologous implants are rigid enough. In cadaveric tests in our lab, all materials from plastics, bone, wood and metals seem equivalent. For low frequencies, even viscous ointment-like connections seem to deliver reasonable results (unpublished observations).

Mass: The middle ear is dominated by stiffness in low frequencies, and mass has little effect here. Of course, if the mass is very large, the frequencies at which it will have an effect become lower and lower. Experience with reconstruction using the whole incus (mass about 30 mg) shows that even this large mass is acceptable. In cadaveric experiments, we loaded masses up to 55 mg onto a SHOT type prosthesis and found only a small, about 5 dB, reduction in stapes velocity above 4 kHz [13] (Fig. 2). Others have found similar small effects from loading masses onto the natural ossicles [14].

Another reason for desiring low mass is the stability of the prosthesis in response to high acceleration forces, such as head trauma. The inertia of heavier prostheses may displace them more than light ones. In unpublished observations, we have found that light titanium prostheses do not displace even up to 5–7 g accelerations. Titanium is desirable in having high rigidity with low mass, but is difficult to shape easily.

Prosthesis Head Size: Because the TM breaks up into smaller vibrating units at higher frequencies, the head size of the prosthesis has to be large enough that it does not just sample a single node on the TM, which may have resonances of its own. The malleus to some extent does this naturally by averaging over the whole TM. Beyond this, large prosthesis head sizes will sample more of the TM, but will also stiffen the TM and may change its impedance matching to air. We com-

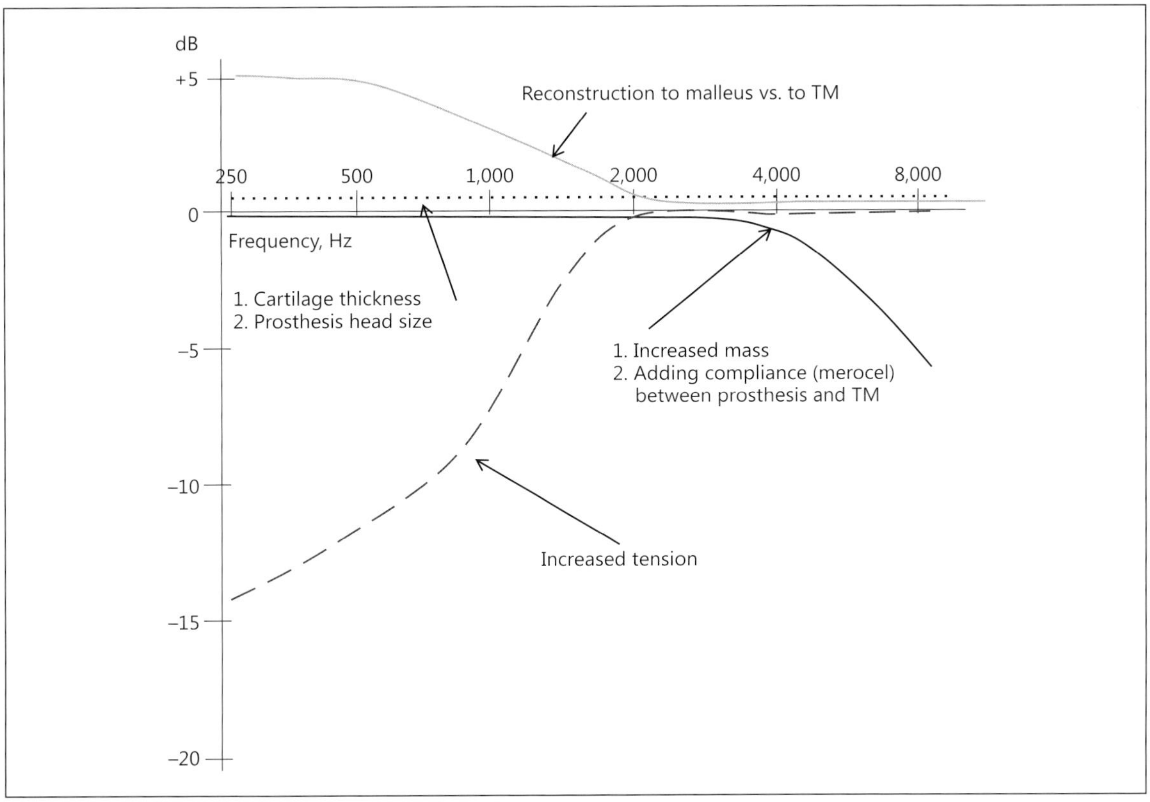

Fig. 2. Summary of effects of different parameter changes on vibration transmission to the stapes, based on our work on (a) increased prosthesis tension which affects the lower frequencies greatly, (b) increased mass which affects the higher frequencies modestly, (c) reconstruction to the malleus versus reconstruction to the TM which improves the lower frequencies modestly, (d) interface between the prosthesis and the TM adding a compliance can affect higher frequencies, (e) prosthesis head size and (f) cartilage thickness between the prosthesis and TM (unpublished data), both of which have little effect.

pared [15] SHOT prosthesis head sizes of 4 × 4, 4 × 3 and 3 × 2 mm in temporal bones with little difference found in the stapes responses (Fig. 2). These sizes encompass most of the sizes of commercial prostheses. There is little need to use a large head size, which is more difficult to place, when a smaller head size is easier to work with.

Placement of Prosthesis

Reconstruct to Malleus or to TM? Clinically, there are so many variables in play that it is difficult to determine if there is a mechanical advantage in reconstructing to the malleus instead of to the TM, with some series showing an advantage, and others no effect.

The malleus may provide some pressure gain through the catenary lever effect [16, 17], though this is controversial there may be some advantage in its utilization. Reconstructing to the malleus, however, means more angulation, a worse force vector and more of a rotational vector (Fig. 1).

We compared [18] reconstruction from the malleus (SHOM) to that from the TM (SHOT), and found a slight (about 5dB) advantage in the malleus reconstruction below 2 kHz (Fig. 2). However, differing tension effects in the 2 types of reconstruction may have contaminated this result. Shimizu and Goode [19] tried to remove the tension effects by using a SHOM reconstruction and then taking out the malleus and placing the prosthesis to the same position on the TM. They found little difference in the results.

Another point of controversy is where to connect on the malleus. Below 1 kHz, the umbo has higher vibration amplitudes [20] but it requires greater angulation to reach and has an unstable geometry. Also, experiments have not shown any advantage in reconstructing to the umbo versus the mid-manubrium [14], whereas others have actually found worse results in connecting to the umbo at high frequencies. Overall, mid-manubrium seems a reasonable choice for stability and function. The malleus at high frequencies also exhibits translational movements, in addition to rotational ones, and the short process is not a low amplitude node for the translational movements as it is for rotational movements. Malleus rotation posteriorly may add to stabilization of the prosthesis, but its mechanical effects are largely unknown.

Where to Place on the Footplate? Again, the findings are not clear. Temporal bone studies by Vlaming and Feenstra [21] found little difference in displacement when reconstructing to the anterior versus central footplate. Other studies have clearly found increased volume velocity of displacement by reconstructing to the centre of the footplate. The posterior position seems to be the worst [22]. In general, reconstruction to the center is advocated.

Reconstruct to Stapes Head or to Footplate? Leaving aside other factors affecting function, especially stability issues, there is conflicting literature as to whether reconstruction to the stapes head (SHOM, FOM) results in better hearing than reconstruction to the footplate (SHOT, FOT). The majority of the literature favors reconstruction to the stapes head if such an arrangement is possible [1]. There is, however, no a-priori mechanical reason for this, except that it is easier to constrain rotation movements on the capitulum than on the footplate. Clinical results may also reflect increased pathology when the reconstruction has to be to the footplate.

In a study where we compared reconstruction from the TM to the stapes head (SHOT) with reconstruction from the TM to the footplate (FOT) in temporal bones [23] there was little difference in the resulting stapes vibrations. In this kind of reconstruction, because it is mostly perpendicular, the force vectors are similar for the FOT and the SHOT. If, however, reconstructing to the malleus, then a SHOM (i.e., stapes head to malleus) has a larger angulation than a FOM. In comparing these SHOM/FOM reconstructions, Murugasu et al. [24] found about a 6 dB advantage in going to the footplate versus the stapes head, although their SHOM prosthesis did not have any design to engage the stapes and may have exhibited excessive rotational movements. There is no convincing evidence to suggest that one type of reconstruction to stapes head or to the footplate is more efficient than the other.

What Tension Should the Prosthesis be Under? We have consistently found tension to have one of the largest effects of any factor tested in reducing low frequency results. Below 2 kHz, excessive tension causes drops in the order of 10–15 dB. This may be due to stiffening the TM, the annular ligament, or both. In this lower frequency region, the ear is dominated by stiffness, so this effect is not too surprising. We have shown this effect for reconstructions to the TM (SHOT) [25] and to the malleus (SHOM) [18]. Others have reported very similar findings [21, 26, 27], consistently showing drops below 1–2 kHz with increased tension.

Clinically, it is difficult to adjust the tension in SHOT or FOT reconstructions, as the TM or reconstruction is laid back down over the prosthesis, but it can be modulated in SHOM or FOM reconstructions if the malleus is still robust. Sometimes tension is also needed for stability. We would recommend the minimum tension needed for stability.

What Should be Placed in the Interface with the TM? Many otologists prefer to cover allografts with cartilage as this reduces the extrusion rate and prevents the TM from retracting around the prosthesis. This cartilage can be varied in its thickness and in its dimensions. Other materials could also be placed here if they gave some mechanical advantage, for example, bone, fascia, fat or other material that might allow for expansion and compression as the position of the TM varied with middle ear pressure. In fact, interestingly, Yamada and Goode [26] report that spongy material at the TM-prosthesis interface could be used as a tension regulating device mitigating the effects of longer prostheses.

We investigated this interface with different sized cartilage pieces and found that smaller cartilage grafts gave better low frequency responses, probably because they did not distort the conical shape of the TM and cause increased stiffness of the TM [28]. We also found little difference in putting glass, cartilage or soft spongy material at this interface, except at frequencies above 4 kHz, where spongy material tended to cause a drop in transmission. In unpublished results, we have also found that the thickness of the cartilage at this interface had little or no effect on vibration transmission to the stapes.

Shimizu and Goode [19] performed similar experiments and reported similar results in that larger cartilage pieces showed larger drops in the stapes vibrations, particularly in the lower frequencies. They report better results at high frequencies with the largest cartilage pieces, which differs from our results and is not in keeping with the previously reported mechanics of the middle ear.

In a more recent study [27], Ulku et al. [27] found that small and large cartilage covers over a SHOT-type prosthesis had little effect on low frequencies, but used a cartilage of 8 mm^2 as their small cartilage and 16 mm^2 as their large size, a difference that is unlikely to increase tension in the TM. They did, however, find that larger cartilage pieces reduced high frequency responses, which they ascribe to a mass effect.

We would recommend, if cartilage is needed to prevent extrusion, that it be approximately the same size as the head of the prosthesis. Larger pieces of cartilage are, however, often used to prevent retraction pockets in the posterior tympanic membrane and this should also be considered when deciding how large the cartilage graft should be.

Surgical Handling

The ideal prostheses should be ergonomic, and easy to place and revise. This can mean different things to different surgeons, but the following are the author's preferences. A perforated head is desirable, as it means that the stem is visible as the prosthesis is placed. A smaller, conformable head, that is, no larger than 4 mm diameter maximum is easier to conform to any remaining TM. A light prosthesis is easier to pick and place with a sucker; however, if it is too light, it is likely to stick to blood and saline and be difficult to manipulate. A prosthesis with a lower centre of gravity is more likely to stay stable after placement, and not tip intra-operatively, as is a prosthesis with a broader base on the stem. An off-center prosthesis is easier to place without hitting the posterior wall. An easily modifiable prosthesis means that the head angle be tilted to shape to TM variables, and there are a few prostheses that try to allow expansion or contraction of the prosthesis for exact fit (e.g., by placing an "S" bend in the shaft that can be opened or compressed). Most prostheses have some kind of sizing system, either with dummies or with measuring rods. While it is ideal, in terms of reducing inventory, to have just one prosthesis that can be configured to different sizes, in practice, this has to be balanced with how "fiddly" it is to modify and change the size of the prosthesis.

Other Issues

Adapting to Static Forces: Ideally, the prosthesis would be able to adapt to changing middle ear pressures. If the TM is lateralized or medialized,

Lloyd SKW, Donnelly NP (eds): Advances in Hearing Rehabilitation.
Adv Otorhinolaryngol. Basel, Karger, 2018, vol 81, pp 24–31 (DOI: 10.1159/000485587)

Advances in the Field of Bone Conduction Hearing Implants

R.W.J. McLeod[a] · J.F. Culling[a] · D. Jiang[b]

[a]School of Psychology, Cardiff University, Tower Building, Cardiff, and [b]St Thomas' Hearing Implant Centre, St Thomas' Hospital, Guy's and St Thomas' NHS Foundation Trust, London, UK

Abstract

The number of marketed bone-conduction hearing implants (BCHIs) has been steadily growing, with multiple percutaneous devices and transcutaneous devices now available. However, studies assessing efficacy often have small sample sizes and employ different assessment methodologies. Thus, there is a paucity of evidence to guide clinicians to the most appropriate device for each patient. This paper outlines audiological guidelines for the latest devices, as well as research from the most up-to-date clinical trials. We also outline the evidence base for some potentially contentious issues in the field of bone conduction, including bilateral fitting of BCHIs in those with bilateral conductive hearing loss as well as the use of BCHIs in single-sided deafness (SSD). Bilateral fitting of BCHIs have been found to significantly increase the hearing thresholds in quiet and improve sound localization, but to give limited benefits in background noise. Studies conducted via multiple assessment questionnaires have found strong evidence of subjective benefits for the use of BCHIs in SSD. However, there is little objective evidence of benefit for SSD patients from sound localization and speech in noise tests.

Introduction

Per-Ingvar Brånemark's 1960 discovery that titanium could be reliably osseointegrated was crucial in the development of dental implants, and also spawned the development of the majority of modern bone-conduction hearing implants (BCHIs) [1]. In 1977, a collaboration made up of Sahlgrenska University Hospital, Chalmers University of Technology and Brånemark Osseointegration Center started the design of the first BCHI [2]. This design consisted of a titanium screw, percutaneous abutment and transducer/sound processor. It had many advantages over its predecessors, including improved transmission of sound (particularly, high frequencies) and elimination of discomfort occurring due to pressure on the skin via Softband devices [3]. Between 1985 (when the first 10 cases were reported by Håkansson [2]) and 2014, there have been approximately 150,000 patients treated with osseointegrated devices [4], with 6,000–7,000 of those performed within the United Kingdom [5].

This paper summarizes the audiological benefits and patient outcomes related to the latest available devices. Additionally, the latest evidence for the use of BCHIs in single-sided deafness (SSD) as well as indications for the appropriateness of bilateral fitting of BCHIs in conductive hearing loss (CHL) will also be discussed.

Device Categorization

Since the original BCHI design, a number of different devices have been marketed but the focus of this paper will be on currently available devices. They can be categorized into 2 main groups: skin-drive and direct-drive devices. Direct-drive devices include products such as the Bone Anchored Hearing Aid (BAHA; Cochlear Bone Anchored Solutions), Ponto (Oticon Medical) and the Bonebridge (Vibrant MED-EL, Innsbruck, Australia). These devices vibrate the skull via direct contact with the bone. Direct-drive devices can be subdivided into: percutaneous devices, where an abutment is used (such as the BAHA and Ponto) and active transcutaneous devices, where the transducer is implanted (such as the Bonebridge). Skin-drive devices, including the Sophono and BAHA Attract, do not have a continuous link with the bone as vibrations are transmitted through the skin to an implanted magnet instead.

Direct-Drive Devices

Cochlear Bone Anchored Solutions' current designs comprise of BAHA 5, BAHA 3 Power and Cordelle II. The BAHA 5 audiological fitting range can compensate for an average of 45 dB bone conduction thresholds across 0.5, 1, 2 and 3 kHz. In comparison, the BAHA 3 Power thresholds can be up to 55 dB. The Cordelle II, which uses a body-worn sound processor, is appropriate for thresholds up to 65 dB over the same frequency range. A single-blinded study, comparing the BAHA 5 to previous generations of processors, found that 9 out of 10 patients rated speech understanding and sound quality good, with 7 out of 10 choosing the latest processor over its predecessors. This shows that improvements in device design are producing noticeable patient benefits [6]. Additionally, a postal questionnaire completed by 227 patients from the Birmingham BCHI program, found that 79.3% of respondents preferred BCHIs over conventional hearing aids or Softband in quiet, and 59.2% in noise [7].

Oticon Medicals' percutaneous bone conduction hearing systems are the Ponto Plus and Ponto Plus Power. Recommended audiological fitting ranges for the Ponto Plus and Ponto Plus Power are that pure conductive and mixed hearing losses do not exceed an average bone conduction threshold of over 45 and 55 dB, respectively. A small study of 12 patients by Olsen et al. [8] compared user preferences between the BP100 BAHA and the Ponto Pro. Both devices have now been upgraded by their respective manufacturers and thus the study's conclusions may no longer be valid. However, the Ponto Pro speech intelligibility was rated higher than the BP100, with 8 of 12 subjects preferring the Ponto Pro overall.

The Bonebridge (Vibrant MED-EL, Innsbruck, Australia) consists of an external sound processor and an internal bone conduction implant (BCI). The BCI has been conditionally certified for magnetic resonance imaging up to 1.5 Tesla and is approved for use in children 5 years or older. The sound processor is worn externally and attached via a variable strength magnet to the patient's head. The BCI includes a floating mass transducer that produces mechanical vibrations transferred to the mastoid bone via 2 cortical screws. Combining audiological results from 45 patients in 4 different studies, there was a mean 29.4 dB gain in aided versus unaided pure tone audiogram results [9–12]. Ihler et al.'s [12] study of 6 patients found that there was a mean improvement of 36.1 in the Glasgow benefit inventory (GBI) postoperatively.

Skin-Drive Devices

The Sophono implant (Medtronic) comprises of 2 magnets encased in a titanium frame. These are secured via 5 screws to the temporal bone after drilling a bony well for the frame to sit in. No percutaneous abutment is present and sound is instead transferred via transcutaneous energy transfer, which is designed to minimize the attenuation caused by the skin between the implant and processor (attached via magnetic attraction) [13]. Studies of twenty patients with congenital unilateral and bilateral canal atresia, have evaluated outcomes from the Sophono device and found that free-field pure tone audiometry (PTA) increased by 28.6 dB [14]. There was also a 61.6% improvement in free-field speech testing (at 65 dB). A case series of 18 patients found that audiological benefits were greatest for those with bilateral CHL (21.9 dB), in comparison to those with a mixed hearing loss who had a relatively moderate gain of 5.5 dB [15].

The BAHA Attract system uses the same titanium implant as the percutaneous system, but instead of an abutment, a magnetic disk is attached subcutaneously. The external sound processor is then attached via the magnet. The recommended maximum bone conduction threshold is 30 dB for the Attract system. A multicenter case series of 27 patients fitted with the Attract system (17 with CHL, 10 with SSD), found a 17.9 dB improvement in PTA in those with CHL, and a 19.1 dB improvement in patients with SSD (although the non-test ear was blocked) [16]. No significant difference was found in PTA when compared to Softband. However, speech understanding in noise was found to improve by 15 dB over the unaided condition and 3.8 dB compared to Softband testing. The abbreviated profile of hearing aid benefit questionnaire showed significant improvements in the background noise domain, the reverberation domain as well as the global score. Two of the 27 patients reported mild/moderate pain after a long period of use, and 4 had mild erythema over the magnet site which resolved over time (one requiring a weaker magnet).

Device Selection

There are multiple factors which need to be considered when selecting an appropriate device (in consultation with the patients). Surgical aspects such as the quality of bone, mastoid size as well as the surgical time and difficulties should all be considered. Poor bone quality leaves patients with an increased risk of failure [17]. While a small mastoid size may mean implantation with a device such as the Bonebridge is not appropriate, especially in children. Preoperative CT planning with 3D reconstruction to assess if implantation is possible (which can be mastoid or retrosigmoid) is recommended for Bonebridge. The length and difficulty of the procedure is a further factor where Oticon's minimally invasive Ponto surgery has shortened and simplified percutaneous fitting considerably. Patient acceptability is an additional major factor which takes into account aesthetics where transcutaneous devices are generally preferred; and cleaning and care of an abutment where relatively high proportions of patients feel this is an issue [7]. Finally, the audiological outcomes are of importance, with current transcutaneous devices often lacking the power of percutaneous devices. Hol et al. [18] found that hearing thresholds were better via the percutaneous BAHA Divo when compared to the transcutaneous Sophono and Briggs et al. [16] failed to find a significant improvement in speech thresholds in quiet with the use of BAHA attract when compared to Softband.

Bilateral versus Unilateral Fitting in Bilateral Conductive Hearing Loss

Binaural hearing relies on the separation of inputs to each cochlea, which facilitates interaural time differences for low frequencies and interaural level differences for high frequencies, produced by head-shadow [19]. However, vibrations from one BCHI travel not only to the ipsilateral cochlea but also to the contralateral cochlea. The universal transmission through the skull bone, which is successfully used to benefit patients with SSD, limits the ability of the auditory system to process binaural information potentially due to the interaction of the vibration waveform arriving to each cochlea in its relative phase and amplitude, and it is often used as a reason for unilateral fitting [20]. However, bilateral BCHIs have been shown to have many advantages, both via objective audiological outcomes and subjective measures.

Audiological Outcomes of Bilateral and Unilateral BCHIs

Bilateral BCHIs have been shown to produce improvements in speech reception thresholds (SRTs) in quiet of 4–5.4 dB when compared to unilateral BCHI fitting [21–23], with similar improvements also identified for tone reception thresholds in quiet [21, 24]. This benefit appears to derive from the increased bone vibration generated by 2 devices working together. Evidence of benefit when listening to speech in noise is clear, but situation dependent. Bilateral BCHIs are advantageous when noise is diffuse, with a 2.8 dB speech-to-noise ratio (SNR) improvement when compared to unilateral BCHI fitting [21]. For a single localized noise source, the benefits of head shadow sometimes occur for the unilateral BCHI control group as well as the bilateral group. So, when noise is presented to the aided side (in the unilateral group), the reported advantages of bilateral fitting are 2.5 [23] and 3.1 [21] dB SNR, but, if noise comes from the unaided side, bilateral benefits are reduced to 0.8 dB [23] and –1 dB [21] SNR.

Binaural masking level difference (BMLD) results (which are a reflection of the ability to perform binaural processing of interaural time differences) are mixed. Air conduction BMLD results are in the range of 11 ± 2 dB in normal hearing subjects [25], but Priwin et al. [21] found no benefit and Bosman et al. [23] found only a 6–6.6 dB BMLD at 125–500 Hz with no benefit at higher frequencies in bilateral BAHA users. Despite limited BMLD results, improvements in sound localization with bilateral BCHIs over unilateral fitting are consistent. Sound localization when using unilateral BCHIs has been found to be extremely poor with significant improvements following bilateral fitting [21, 23, 24]. Snik et al. [26] identified a 53% improvement in sound localization over the unilateral condition.

Subjective Outcomes of Bilateral and Unilateral BCHIs

Bilateral BCHIs consistently show significant improvements in the quality of life (QOL), with a 20-patient study finding a 38-point increase in the Glasgow Children's Benefit Inventory [27]. A further study of 93 bilateral BCHI patients using the GBI found that benefit scores were significantly higher than in a unilateral BCHI population and that scores were similar to those measured after cochlear implantation [28].

Bilateral versus Unilateral Fitting Summary

There is good evidence that bilateral BCHI fitting improves speech/tone thresholds, both in quiet and in noise, as well as sound localization via the addition of interaural cues. Subjective outcomes have shown significant improvements in GBI, although the second BCHI increased it less than the first [29]. Future developments could include the use of phase inversion between BCHIs which, at low frequencies, has the ability to increase signal summation [30]. Additionally, it may be possible to develop a cross-talk cancellation technology, allowing sound reaching the contralateral cochlea to be cancelled by an out-of-phase signal from the contralateral BCHI, thus allowing improved stereo separation and the restoration of interaural cues [31].

Bone Conduction Devices in SSD

There are thought to be approximately 9,000 new diagnoses of SSD in the UK each year, with 24% of sufferers having to give up work as a result [32].

Commonly reported issues from SSD patients include social exclusion associated with difficulties keeping up with group conversations, dangers as a pedestrian as well as increased problems with communication in the workplace [32]. Since sufferers have only one working cochlea, they cannot process any interaural cues and so lack the ability to derive any of the normal benefits of binaural processing, such as improved sound localization and understanding of speech in background noise [33]. Treatment options of SSD include education related to the best sitting positions in noisy environments to make the most use of monaural clues. Hearing devices are also available in the form of a Contralateral Routing of Signal (CROS) hearing aid and a BCHI. Several countries have also approved cochlear implantation as a treatment option [34].

In 2002, the FDA approved the use of BCHI for SSD. Since then, there has been an increasing number of patients being treated with this method [37]. Although binaural hearing cannot be restored, the BCHI makes use of the relatively limited transcranial attenuation to allow sound from the deaf side to be transferred to the contralateral side. This aims to improve the detection of sound when the sound is laterally projected to the deaf side [38].

Patients with congenital SSD are an important subgroup who are at a greater risk of learning problems at school when compared to those with normal hearing [35]. Prevalence rates of congenital SSD are estimated to be in the region of 0.1% [36]. It has been theorized that these patients may not benefit as much from treatment with either BCHI or CROS, because such patients have always relied on a monaural strategy of processing pinna-induced spectral-shape cues. However, research has failed to find significant evidence for this hypothesis, instead discovering that localization ability in patients with SSD is dependent on high-frequency cues [34].

Despite much published literature, evidence for the benefit of BCHI in SSD is inconsistent with most subjective studies showing benefit, while most objective studies do not. A recent review concluded that there was a lack of high level evidence for both BCHI and CROS in SSD [39]. A summary of both subjective and objective results is presented in Table 1.

In the subjective studies, measures such as the abbreviated profile of hearing aid benefit have been widely used. This comprises assessment in a number of domains including: ease of communication, background noise, reverberation, aversion to loud noise, as well as a global score. Studies consistently found significant improvements in ease of communication and in the background noise domains. In contrast, scores tended to be poorer in the assessment of aversion to loud noise [40–45]. The single-sided deafness questionnaire is a further commonly used assessment tool which found that the majority of patients use their devices between 4 and 7 h a day and that there was a perceived benefit in QOL and in hearing (particularly, in quiet) [40, 43, 44].

Several objective studies have investigated BCHI via the use of hearing in noise testing, the majority of which have found benefits only when speech is directed to the deaf ear. In this experimental configuration, there is an improvement in thresholds due to compensation of the head shadow effect by BCHI. In the converse condition, however, where speech is directed to the hearing ear and noise to the deaf ear, the hearing threshold worsens due to head shadow being compensated for [40–42, 45, 46]. Thus, overall there is no benefit. Lin et al. [45] reported that the increases in the beneficial condition were greater than the decreases in the detrimental condition, but these differences were not significant. One study of twenty-one patients with SSD and contralateral hearing loss did find significant improvements in speech recognition in both quiet and noise. Since the benefit in noise occurred regardless of a spatial separation between speech and noise, this benefit must be related to improvement in the stimulus audibility, and so might not be sustained if the stimulus were presented at a higher sound level.

Table 1. Summary of study findings investing the use of BCHI for SSD treatment

Authors	Objective measures			Subjective measures					Study conclusions
	HINT	SRT	SL	APHAB	SSDQ	GHABP	SSQ	GBI	
Lin et al. [45]	×*		×	✓					Benefit
Linstrom et al. [40]	×*			✓	✓				Benefit
Yuen et al. [41]	×†			✓		✓			Benefit
Arndt et al. [48]			×				×		No benefit
Dumper et al. [42]	×			✓			×		Limited benefit
Martin et al. [46]	×						×	×	No benefit
Wazen et al. [49]	✓‡							✓	Benefit
Gluth et al. [43]				✓	✓	✓			Benefit
Hol et al. [44]			×	✓	✓		✓		Benefit
Bovo et al. [38]		×							No benefit
Pai et al. [37]							✓		Benefit

* Benefits only when noise front and speech lateralized to bad ear, † Benefits were found; however, HINT only performed with speech from deaf side, ‡ Study was of SSD patients with contralateral hearing loss. HINT, hearing in noise testing; SRT, speech reception threshold; SL, source localization; APHAB, abbreviated profile of hearing aid benefit; SSDQ, single-sided deafness questionnaire; GHABP, Glasgow hearing aid benefit profile; SSQ, speech, spatial and qualities of hearing scale; GBI, Glasgow benefit inventory.

Future devices may be able to improve hearing in noise testing in BCHI users via communication with an additional microphone on the normal hearing side. Scene classification technology, currently used to benefit cochlear implant users [47], could then adaptively turn the BCHI on and off depending on how favorable the signal-to-noise ratio is on the deaf side.

Conclusion

The introduction of the Sophono, Bonebridge and BAHA Attract have identified a trend towards transcutaneous devices, with manufacturers of percutaneous devices such as the BAHA 5 and Ponto Plus creating sound processors with smaller profiles [4]. These innovations recognize the drive for devices to require less maintenance and be more aesthetically acceptable to patients. The current amplification ability of transcutaneous devices often, however, falls short of the percutaneous competition. This indicates that percutaneous devices are potentially more appropriate when a patient has a significant sensorineural hearing loss component. For those with bilateral CHL, bilateral fitting of a BCHI may be appropriate, with studies showing increases in QOL measures and benefits in sound localization and thresholds in quiet. Additionally, patients with SSD find significant benefits in multiple subjective measures. Evidence for objective audiological benefits was limited with benefits only in specific experimental configurations and when the contralateral ear had suboptimal hearing thresholds. The BCHI continues to be a highly valuable treatment option for patients. Smaller visible size, combined with improved sound processing and greater power, imply that future patients will have even higher patient satisfaction.

Disclosure Statement

R.W.J.M. has received research funding from Cochlear Bone Anchored Solutions. Other authors report no conflicts of interest.

Table 1. Active middle ear implant score (aMEI-score) for aural atresia

Oval window subscore[1]	OW ossified		0	
	Stapes present	Stapes corridor ≤5 mm	2	
		Stapes corridor >5 mm	4	
		Stapes corridor >10 mm	6	
	Stapes absent	OW corridor ≤5 mm	0	
		OW corridor >5 mm	2	
		OW corridor >10 mm	4	0–6[7]
Round window subscore[2]	RW ossified		0	
	RW open	Anterior RW corridor ≤5 mm	0	
		Anterior RW corridor >5 mm	2	
		Anterior RW corridor >10 mm	4	
		Posterior RW corridor ≤5 mm	0	
		Posterior RW corridor >5 mm	1	
		Posterior RW corridor >10 mm	2	0–4[7]
Middle ear pneumatization[3]	Hypoplastic or opacified middle ear cavity		0	
	Aerated middle ear cavity		2	0–2[7]
Mastoid pneumatization[4]	Ebonized mastoid		0	
	Opacified mastoid		1	
	Aerated mastoid		2	0–2[7]
Tegmen mastoideum[5]	Inferior displaced		0	
	Normal		1	0–1[7]
Facial nerve at oval window[6]	Inferior displaced		0	
	Normal		1	0–1[7]
Total	(16–13 easy, 12–9 moderate, 8–5 difficult and 4–0 high risk)			

[1] An open oval window (OW) is defined as a definite cleft of normal size in the otic capsule. Windows <1 mm or dense bone receive no point. A present stapes is defined as near-normal shaped ossicle with an intact arch and head. A malformed or absent stapes receives no points. If the oval window is open and the stapes present, use the stapes corridor: A line is drawn from the head of stapes along the anterior limit of the third segment of the facial nerve, and the distance from the anterior limitation to this line is measured. If the oval window is open and the stapes absent, use the oval window corridor: The corridor is determined in the axial plane that captures the center line. A line is drawn from the posterior limit of the oval window niche along the anterior limit of the third segment of the facial nerve, and the distance from the anterior limitation to this line is measured. [2] An open round window (RW) is defined as a definite cleft of normal size in the otic capsule. Windows of <1 mm or dense bone receive no point. If the round window is open, the anterior round window corridor is determined in the axial plane that captures the center line. A line is drawn from the posterior limit of the round window niche along the anterior limit of the third segment of the facial nerve, and the distance from the anterior limitation to this line is measured. The posterior round window corridor is determined in the axial plane that captures the center line. A line is drawn from the anterior limit of the round window niche along the posterior limit of the third segment of the facial nerve, and the distance from the sigmoid sinus to this line is measured. [3] A pneumatized middle ear is defined as an aerated middle ear cavity of normal or reduced size. An opacified middle ear is defined as a fluid- or soft tissue-filled cavity of normal or reduced size. A middle ear is hypoplastic if its size is less than 30% of a normal cavity independent of aeration. [4] A pneumatized mastoid is defined as an aerated antrum and beyond. Patients with a pneumatized mastoid have aerated cells lateral to the inner atresia plate and labyrinth, with extension into the mastoid. An opacified mastoid is defined as a fluid- or soft tissue-filled mastoid. An ebonized mastoid is defined as a sclerotic or ossified mastoid. [5] The tegmen mastoideum is defined as inferiorly displaced if it extends down to the axial plane of the lateral semicircular canal. [6] The tympanic segment of the facial nerve is defined as inferiorly displaced if it extends down to the inferior limit of the oval window in the coronal plane. [7] Highest value of the previous column. Patients with closed windows receive 0 points independent of the corridor size.

Soft Tissue Approach

The technique presented here – the "posterior atresia incision" – allows wide access to the lateral skull base with good exposure of the atresia plate [28]. The technique works with any of the following presented hearing implants. Wound healing leaves behind a hairline scar at an adequate distance from the final ear position.

The final position of the ear is calculated based on the size required, the distance to the nose, eye and the hairline [29]. The average size of the outer ear is 30–35 × 60–65 mm. The base of the lobule is leveled with the nasal base. The top edge of the helix is leveled with the top edge of the eyebrow. The longitudinal axis of the ear is parallel to the bridge of the nose. The distance between the ear and the lateral orbit is 60–70 mm. The important vascular structures (superficial temporal and postauricular artery) are marked. The incision line is positioned 15–20 mm posterior to the anticipated position of the auricle and performed directly through all layers. The periosteum is temporarily sutured to the skin to avoid any shearing of the layers. The atresia plane is widely exposed through a subperiosteal preparation. This technique is illustrated in Figure 1.

Active Middle Ear Implants

These implants have the microphone, processor and energy supply in the external part, which transmits the signal to the internal part. The skin remains intact. The internal part transmits the signal to the transducer in the middle ear. The transducer can be coupled to the stapes (most favorable option), the remnant chain or round window membrane. Coupling to the remnant chain should be carefully selected as the ossicles tend to re-ossify with the cavity wall. Additionally, the incudostapedial joint often only has a fibrous connection, which attenuates the sound transmission [29]. If the stapes are selected for coupling, the fused malleus-incus-complex is removed. Coupling to the round window is equally effective and may be used in the absence of a functional ossicular chain. The transducer is stabilized with cartilage. However, the approach to the round window niche is much more sophisticated and depends on the position of the facial nerve relative to the round window [23].

To place the transducer, it is necessary to access the middle ear space. There are 2 operative corridors (anterior and posterior) towards the malformed middle ear cavity. The selection is based on the preoperative image analysis. If the target for the transducer placement is the stapes, the anterior corridor should be used because the course of the tympanic and mastoid section of the facial nerve is on average 4 mm more anterior compared to normal ears [3]. To achieve adequate visualization of the head of stapes, the drilling starts far anterior and posterior-superior to the temporomandibular joint [23] (Fig. 2). Working along the tegmen, the lateral semicircular canal and the short process of the incus can be identified. Hence, the atretic bone can be safely removed and the remnant chain exposed.

If the target for transducer placement is the round window, the approach used depends on the position of the facial nerve relative to the round window [23]. Both corridors are possible, and the wider one is selected for implantation. The anterior corridor technique is described above. The posterior corridor technique enters the hypotympanum retrofacially (Fig. 3). The drilling starts with a partial mastoidectomy. After the identification of the lateral semicircular canal and the short process of the incus, the facial nerve and the sigmoid sinus are egg-shelled. These 2 structures determine the limit and angle of the posterior corridor. Finally, the hypotympanum is entered through a retrofacial approach. The niche is enlarged to allow a perpendicular placement of the transducer onto the round window membrane. Couplers and/or cartilage are used to stabilize the transducer.

To date, the active middle ear implant "Vibrant Soundbridge" (MEDEL, Innsbruck,

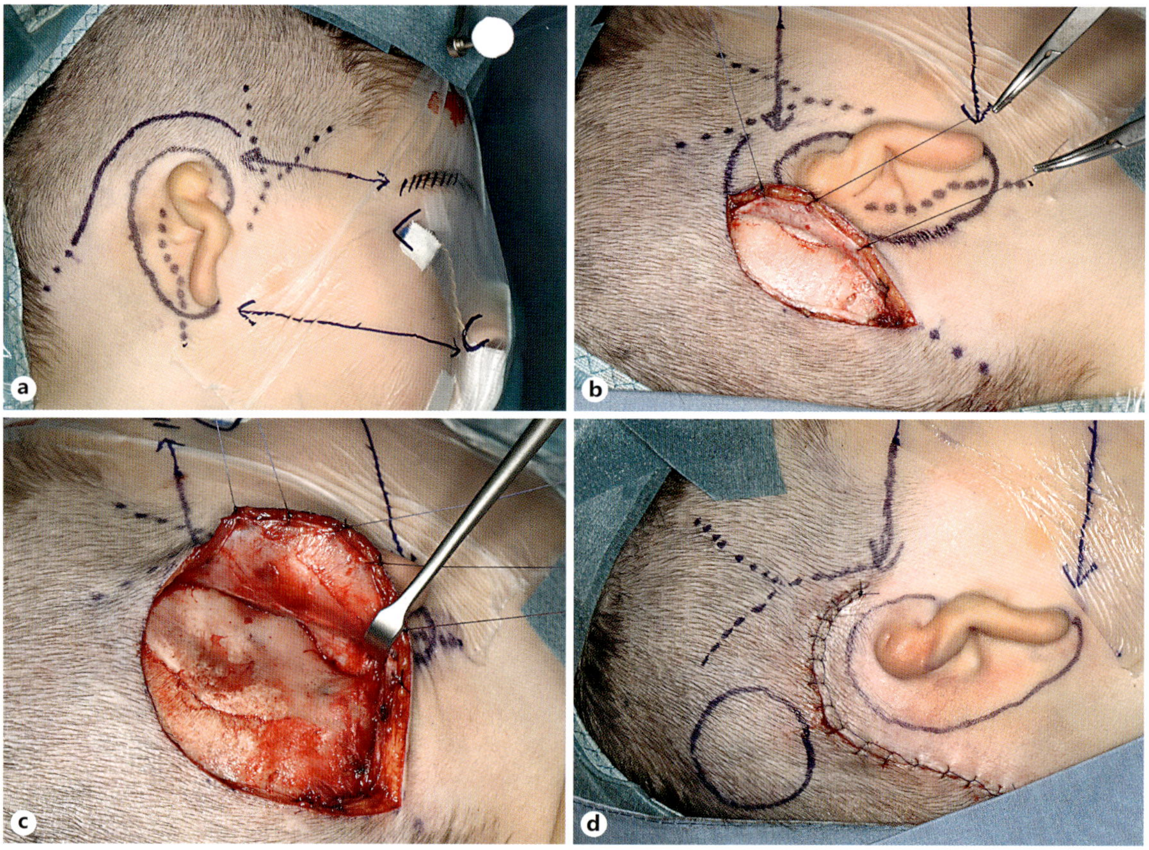

Fig. 1. Posterior atresia incision. **a** The final position of the ear and the vascular structures are marked. The incision line is positioned 15–20 mm posterior to the anticipated position of the auricle. **b** The incision is performed directly through all layers down to the bone, followed by a subperiostal mobilization. To avoid any shearing of the tissue layers, the periosteum is temporarily sutured to the skin. **c** The atresia plane is widely exposed. Mastoid, temporal bone, zygoma and the temporomandibular joint are visualized. **d** The wound is closed in layers and the position of the receiver coil is marked.

Austria) is the only one approved for usage in children and is the most widely used in clinical practice. It has been used for this purpose since 2005 and likely provides the most sophisticated hearing rehabilitation because it is able to selectively stimulate the affected ear.

Active Bone Conduction Implants

These implants have the microphone, processor and energy supply in the external part, which transmits the signal to the internal part. The skin remains intact. The internal part generates mechanical vibration and transduces it through the skull to the cochlea. The transducer sits in a drilled recess in the skull.

The approach to the lateral skull base and exposure of the atretic plane are exactly the same as that for active middle ear implants. The recess for the implant is drilled in the sinodural angle in most cases of aural atresia as this offers the maximum space. However, some contact or indentation of the dura and/or sigmoid sinus is likely in the majority of cases. Thorough preoperative planning of the implant position is essential to

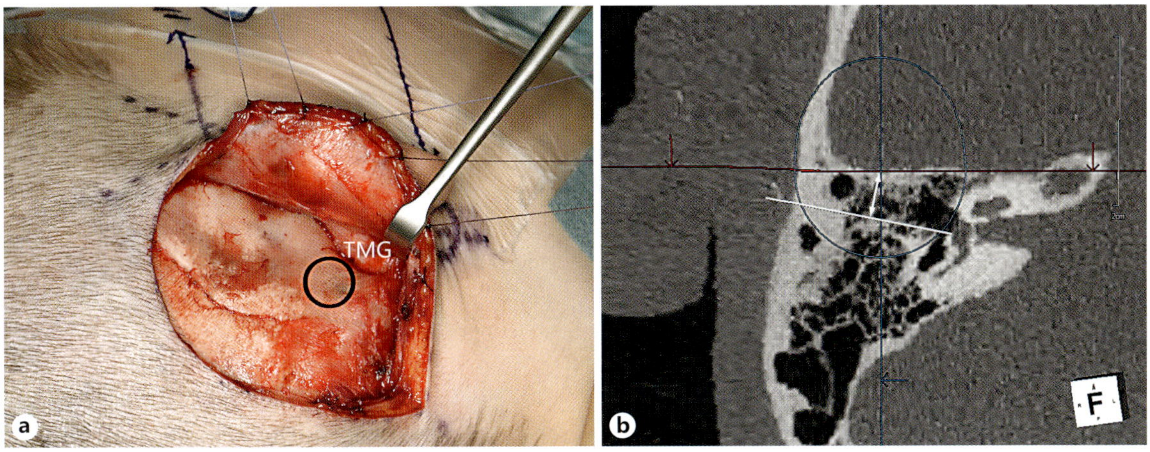

Fig. 2. Anterior operative corridor. This approach is feasible for access to the stapes, oval window and anterior round window. **a** The drilling starts far anterior (black circle), just posterior-superior to temporomandibular joint. **b** The working channel and the vision are limited by the axis (white line) from the target (here the oval window) along the anterior facial nerve and the width to the middle cranial fossa (white arrow) as shown on a coronal CT of the atretic ear. For details, refer to Frenzel et al. [23]. Reproduced with permission.

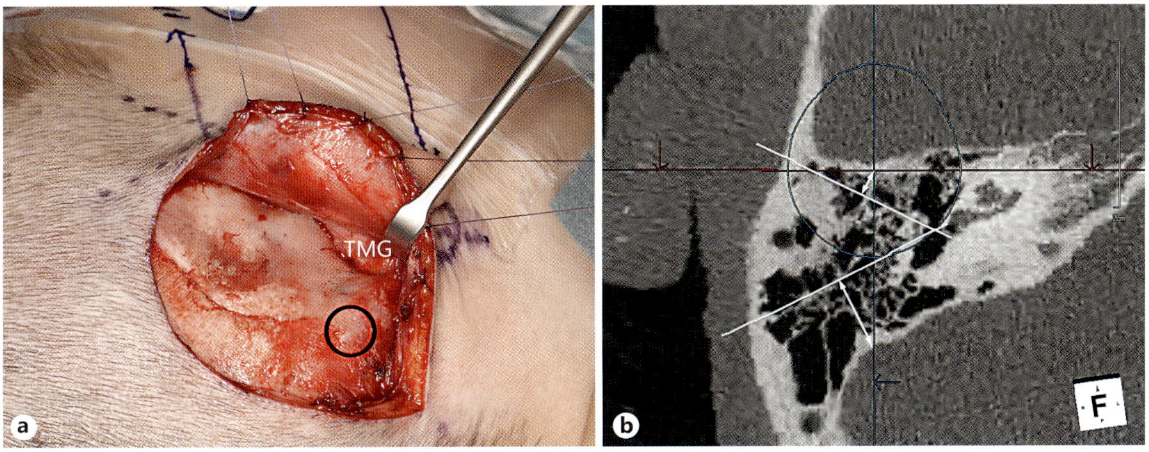

Fig. 3. Posterior operative corridor. This approach is feasible for a retrofacial access to the round window. **a** The drilling starts with a partial mastoidectomy (black circle). **b** The working channel and the vision are limited by the axis (white line) from the target (here the round window) along the posterior facial nerve and the width to the posterior brain fossa (white arrow) as shown on a coronal CT of the atretic ear. For details, refer to Frenzel et al. [23]. Reproduced with permission.

minimize the extent of the indentation. Three-dimensional planning software may be helpful in this respect. Because the skin is very thin in this area, the implant should sit flush with the surface of the bone.

To date, the active bone conduction implant "Vibrant Bonebridge" (MEDEL, Innsbruck, Austria) is the only one approved for use in children. It has been used for this purpose since 2012 and provides reliable hearing rehabilitation. The stimulation within the bone facilitates effective transmission. Like all bone conduction devices, transcranial stimulation of both cochleae is an intrinsic part of the concept.

Passive Bone Conduction Implants

These implants have the microphone, processor, transmitter, transducer and energy supply in the external part, which transmits the signal to a transcutaneous magnet or a percutaneous, osseo integrated abutment. The mechanical vibration travels through the skull to the cochlea. The incision line is 15–20 mm superior-posterior to the anticipated position of the auricle. The lateral skull base does not need to be exposed. These implants have been used for decades and provide a reliable hearing restoration.

There are 2 percutaneous systems available (BAHA Connect, Cochlear, Ltd., Sydney, Australia; Ponto Bone Anchored Hearing System, Oticon Medical, Askim, Sweden). These devices can have problems because the percutaneous screw may be a source of infection and abutment loss. This issue has been addressed by the development of transcutaneous coupling to an implanted magnet. The energy is transmitted through the intact skin by the corresponding internal and external magnets. There are 2 systems available (BAHA Attract, Cochlear, Ltd., Sydney, Australia; Sophono, Medtronic, Minneapolis, MN, USA). These devices provide less gain than the percutaneous devices because the skin absorbs some energy and dampens the transmission. Pressure marks can also occur which can rarely lead to significant skin problems.

Outcome

All hearing implants improve speech perception, speech recognition, signal-to-noise ratio and directional hearing to a varying extent. The active middle ear implant "Vibrant Soundbridge" has proven safety and efficacy in various case series and one prospective multicenter study [30–38]. Word recognition scores over 90% were obtained in all studies. The efficacy did not depend on the severity of the malformation [39]. The active bone conduction implant "Vibrant Bonebridge" has recently also demonstrated safety and comparable efficacy in terms of speech recognition in the first case series when compared to aMEIs [35, 40–42]. The transcutaneous bone conduction devices "BAHA Attract" and "Sophono Alpha" have also demonstrated safety and efficacy in early case series. The audiological outcome, however, seems to be inferior compared to active bone conduction implants or percutaneous bone conduction devices [43–47]. Percutaneous bone conduction devices themselves have proven efficacy in various case series and studies [26]. This recent review [26] additionally emphasizes the superior hearing outcome with implantable hearing aids compared to conventional atresia surgery.

To date, there is a shortage of comparative, prospective studies with standardized outcome measures to adequately distinguish between the different available implants. In general, comparison of outcome measures between existing studies and devices remains quite difficult because of the heterogeneity of speech testing methods.

Conclusion

There is growing evidence that hearing rehabilitation for children with aural atresia should be undertaken as early as possible. This applies to both unilateral and bilateral atresia. In general, hearing implants seem to provide a more stable and more efficient hearing outcome compared to conventional atresia surgery. For selected cases with minor malformations, middle ear reconstruction in combination with tympanoplasty can be a viable option.

The selection of the type of hearing implant depends on the age of the patient and the severity of the malformation. It is assumed that a selective and early stimulation of the cochleae allows the patient to develop true binaural hearing. Hence, an active middle ear implant applied within the first years of life may lead to the most beneficial hearing rehabilitation. Older patients and patients with severe malformations are adequately rehabilitated with one of the available bone conduction devices. To date, however, there are not enough comparative studies to prove this hypothesis and to allow an evidence-based comparison of the different available implants.

References

1 Bartel-Friedrich S: Congenital auricular malformations: description of anomalies and syndromes. Facial Plast Surg 2015; 31:567–580.
2 Goldsztein H, Roberson JB Jr: Anatomical facial nerve findings in 209 consecutive atresia cases. Otolaryngol Head Neck Surg 2013;148:648–652.
3 Takegoshi H, et al: Facial canal anatomy in patients with microtia: evaluation of the temporal bones with thin-section CT. Radiology 2002;225:852–858.
4 Bess FH, Tharpe AM: Unilateral hearing impairment in children. Pediatrics 1984; 74:206–216.
5 Ito K: Can unilateral hearing loss be a handicap in learning? Arch Otolaryngol Head Neck Surg 1998;124:1389–1390.
6 Keller WD, Bundy RS: Effects of unilateral hearing loss upon educational achievement. Child Care Health Dev 1980;6:93–100.
7 Kesser BW, Krook K, Gray LC: Impact of unilateral conductive hearing loss due to aural atresia on academic performance in children. Laryngoscope 2013;123: 2270–2275.
8 Lieu JE: Speech-language and educational consequences of unilateral hearing loss in children. Arch Otolaryngol Head Neck Surg 2004;130:524–530.
9 Kuppler K, Lewis M, Evans AK: A review of unilateral hearing loss and academic performance: is it time to reassess traditional dogmata? Int J Pediatr Otorhinolaryngol 2013;77:617–622.
10 Lieu JE, Tye-Murray N, Fu Q: Longitudinal study of children with unilateral hearing loss. Laryngoscope 2012;122: 2088–2095.
11 Klatte M, Lachmann T, Meis M: Effects of noise and reverberation on speech perception and listening comprehension of children and adults in a classroom-like setting. Noise Health 2010;12:270–282.
12 Gordon KA, Wong DD, Papsin BC: Bilateral input protects the cortex from unilaterally-driven reorganization in children who are deaf. Brain 2013;136: 1609–1625.
13 Kral A, et al: Single-sided deafness leads to unilateral aural preference within an early sensitive period. Brain 2013;136: 180–193.
14 Gordon KA, et al: Use it or lose it? Lessons learned from the developing brains of children who are deaf and use cochlear implants to hear. Brain Topogr 2011; 24:204–219.
15 Moore JK, Linthicum FH Jr: The human auditory system: a timeline of development. Int J Audiol 2007;46:460–478.
16 Gordon KA, Wong DD, Papsin BC: Cortical function in children receiving bilateral cochlear implants simultaneously or after a period of interimplant delay. Otol Neurotol 2010;31:1293–1299.
17 Verhagen CV, et al: The Baha Softband. A new treatment for young children with bilateral congenital aural atresia. Int J Pediatr Otorhinolaryngol 2008;72: 1455–1459.
18 Frenzel H, et al: The Lübeck flowchart for functional and aesthetic rehabilitation of aural atresia and microtia. Otol Neurotol 2012;33:1363–1367.
19 Gray L, Kesser B, Cole E: Understanding speech in noise after correction of congenital unilateral aural atresia: Effects of age in the emergence of binaural squelch but not in use of head-shadow. Int J Pediatr Otorhinolaryngol 2009;73:1281–1287.
20 Arndt S, et al: Cochlear implantation in children with single-sided deafness: does aetiology and duration of deafness matter? Audiol Neurootol 2015;20(suppl 1):21–30.
21 Távora-Vieira D, Rajan GP: Cochlear implantation in children with congenital and noncongenital unilateral deafness: a case series. Otol Neurotol 2015;36:235–239.
22 Jahrsdoerfer RA, et al: Grading system for the selection of patients with congenital aural atresia. Am J Otol 1992;13: 6–12.
23 Frenzel H, et al: Grading system for the selection of patients with congenital aural atresia for active middle ear implants. Neuroradiology 2013;55:895–911.
24 Dazert S, Thomas JP, Volkenstein S: Surgical and technical modalities for hearing restoration in ear malformations. Facial Plast Surg 2015;31:581–586.
25 Roberson JB Jr, et al: Atresia repair before microtia reconstruction: comparison of early with standard surgical timing. Otol Neurotol 2009;30:771–776.
26 Nadaraja GS, et al: Hearing outcomes of atresia surgery versus osseointegrated bone conduction device in patients with congenital aural atresia: a systematic review. Otol Neurotol 2013;34:1394–1399.
27 De la Cruz A, Teufert KB: Congenital aural atresia surgery: long-term results. Otolaryngol Head Neck Surg 2003;129: 121–127.
28 Frenzel H, et al: Application of the Vibrant Soundbridge in bilateral congenital atresia in toddlers. Acta Otolaryngol 2010;130:966–970.
29 Weerda H: Surgery of the Auricle: Tumors-Trauma-Defects-Abnormalities. Weerda, H (ed). Stuttgart, Thieme, 2007.
30 Claros P, Pujol Mdel C: Active middle ear implants: Vibroplasty™ in children and adolescents with acquired or congenital middle ear disorders. Acta Otolaryngol 2013;133:612–619.
31 Colletti L, et al: The floating mass transducer for external auditory canal and middle ear malformations. Otol Neurotol 2011;32:108–115.

32 Frenzel H, et al: Application of the Vibrant Soundbridge to unilateral osseous atresia cases. Laryngoscope 2009;119: 67–74.
33 Frenzel H, et al: The vibrant soundbridge in children and adolescents: Preliminary European multicenter results. Otol Neurotol 2015;36:1216–1222.
34 Hempel JM, Braun T, Berghaus A: [Functional and aesthetic rehabilitation of microtia in children and adolescents]. HNO 2013;61:655–661.
35 Jovankovicova A, et al: Surgery or implantable hearing devices in children with congenital aural atresia: 25 years of our experience. Int J Pediatr Otorhinolaryngol 2015;79:975–979.
36 Lesinskas E, Stankeviciute V, Petrulionis M: Application of the Vibrant Soundbridge middle-ear implant for aural atresia in patients with Treacher Collins syndrome. J Laryngol Otol 2012;126: 1216–1223.
37 Verhaert N, et al: Strategies of active middle ear implants for hearing rehabilitation in congenital aural atresia. Otol Neurotol 2011;32:639–645.
38 Zernotti ME, et al: Vibrant Soundbridge in congenital osseous atresia: multicenter study of 12 patients with osseous atresia. Acta Otolaryngol 2013;133:569–573.
39 Frenzel H: Validation of the aMEI-Score for Selection of Aural Atresia Cases for Active Middle ear Implants [in German] in 85th Annual Meeting of the German Society of Oto-Rhino-Laryngology, Head and Neck Surgery. Dortmund, German Medical Science GMS Publishing House, 2014.
40 Rahne T, et al: Functional results after Bonebridge implantation in adults and children with conductive and mixed hearing loss. Eur Arch Otorhinolaryngol 2015;272:3263–3269.
41 Riss D, et al: Indication criteria and outcomes with the Bonebridge transcutaneous bone-conduction implant. Laryngoscope 2014;124:2802–2806.
42 Sprinzl GM, Wolf-Magele A: The bonebridge bone conduction hearing implant: indication criteria, surgery and a systematic review of the literature. Clin Otolaryngol 2016;41:131–143.
43 Zernotti ME, et al: Comparative outcomes of active and passive hearing devices by transcutaneous bone conduction. Acta Otolaryngol 2016;136: 556–558.
44 Shin JW, et al: Surgical and audiologic comparison between sophono and bone-anchored hearing aids implantation. Clin Exp Otorhinolaryngol 2016;9: 21–26.
45 Nelissen RC, et al: Three-year experience with the Sophono in children with congenital conductive unilateral hearing loss: tolerability, audiometry, and sound localization compared to a bone-anchored hearing aid. Eur Arch Otorhinolaryngol 2016;273:3149–3156.
46 Denoyelle F, et al: Hearing rehabilitation with the closed skin bone-anchored implant Sophono Alpha1: results of a prospective study in 15 children with ear atresia. Int J Pediatr Otorhinolaryngol 2015;79:382–387.
47 Zwartenkot JW, et al: Amplification options for patients with mixed hearing loss. Otol Neurotol 2014;35:221–226.

PD Dr. med. Henning Frenzel
Microtia Germany, Otorhinolaryngology and Facial Plastic Surgery, HNO-Praxis-Lübeck
Schüsselbuden 30/32
DE–23552 Lübeck (Germany)
E-Mail h.frenzel@hno-praxis-luebeck.de

Lloyd SKW, Donnelly NP (eds): Advances in Hearing Rehabilitation.
Adv Otorhinolaryngol. Basel, Karger, 2018, vol 81, pp 43–56 (DOI: 10.1159/000485529)

Hearing Rehabilitation with Active Middle Ear Implants

Neil P. Donnelly[a] • Ronald J.E. Pennings[b, c]

[a]Department of Otolaryngology, Cambridge University Hospitals NHS Foundation Trust, Cambridge, UK; [b]Department of Otorhinolaryngology, Radboud University Medical Center, and [c]Donders Institute for Brain, Cognition and Behaviour, Radboud University, Nijmegen, The Netherlands

Abstract

Hearing implant technology is evolving at a rapid rate and more than ever patients with hearing loss are benefiting from these emerging hearing devices. Active middle ear implants are alternatives to hearing aids and bone conducting devices, offering patients an expanded range in improving their hearing. This chapter looks at the devices currently available, their indications and the literature regarding their outcomes.

Introduction

Hearing loss can be rehabilitated by different types of hearing aids. Conventional acoustic hearing aids (CHA) are most commonly used as they provide excellent amplification for the majority of patients. There are, however, limitations to CHA, including acoustic feedback, distortion, occlusion effect and insufficient gain in patients with severe to profound hearing impairment. Other types of implantable hearing devices have therefore been developed and include bone conduction devices (BCD), active middle ear implants (AMEI), cochlear implants and auditory brainstem implants. These devices aim to restore hearing by interacting with different aspects of the auditory pathway.

Middle ear implants (MEI) are divided into active and passive implants. Passive implants are ossiculoplasty prostheses that attempt to restore middle ear mechanics by coupling the tympanic membrane to remnants of the ossicular chain or cochlea. AMEI are devices placed in the middle ear to amplify hearing. This paper does not review passive implants. Instead, the focus is on AMEI that transduce sound into mechanical energy that drives the ossicular chain or cochlear windows.

AMEI are an alternative to CHA for the rehabilitation of hearing loss. In general, CHA has more advantage than AMEI. CHA have the disadvantage of occluding the external ear canal: this not only leads to autophony but may also give rise to recurrent otitis externa in patients with skin diseases (e.g., psoriasis or eczema). AMEI provide a good alternative in such cases when CHA cannot be used.

Before proceeding, it is important to make a statement on how to report the outcomes

Table 1. Different types of AMEI

Type	Company	Transducer	Fully implantable?	Occlusion effect
Vibrant Soundbridge	MED EL	Electromagnetic	No	No
Carina	Cochlear Limited	Electromechanical	Yes	No
Esteem	Envoy Medical	Piezoelectric	Yes	No

following AMEI placement. Functional gain is often used to report the performance of AMEI. There are, however, several reasons that this is not the ideal means of presenting results in this setting. First, the functional gain is defined as the difference between aided and unaided sound-field thresholds applied in sensorineural hearing loss (SNHL) for devices with linear gain and not for devices that use compression techniques [1]. When compression is used, the measured functional gain is just the gain for low-level sounds and does not represent the gain at normal conversational levels. Secondly, the functional gain is directly influenced by the width of the air-bone gap and therefore it should not be used to evaluate the performance in cases with mixed hearing loss (MHL) or conductive hearing loss (CHL) and only in SNHL. It is, therefore, better to speak about functional improvement and effective gain, defined as the difference between cochlear (bone conduction) thresholds and aided thresholds [2]. Despite the fact that the functional gain is not the best representation of performance for AMEI, an overview of the literature will be presented in this paper including data on functional gain because this term is used in most papers to evaluate performance. For more information on effective gain and maximum power output of different types of auditory implants, which lies outside the scope of this paper, we refer to the informative blog of Snik [2] on this subject.

Three AMEI systems are currently commercially available on the market. These are the Vibrant Soundbridge® (VSB) device (MED-EL, Austria), the fully implantable Carina® (Cochlear Corporation, Australia) device and the fully implantable Esteem® Hearing Implant (Envoy Medical Corporation, USA). Table 1 presents an overview of these devices. The following implants will not be reviewed because they are either under development or no longer available on the market: DACS (Cochlear), MET/Otologics (Cochlear), DACS-PI (Sonova), Rion Device E-type (Japan), TICA (Implex and Tübingen University, Germany), DDHS (Soundtec), SIMEHD (Cleveland, USA), AMEI (Tübingen University, Germany), Ear Lens (EarLens Corp., USA) and MAXUM (Ototronix).

AMEI systems are attached or "coupled" to the ossicles or cochlear windows, this technique has come to be known as vibroplasty. Vibroplasty is defined as the treatment for hearing loss via vibratory stimulation in the middle ear. Beleites et al. [3] introduced a vibroplasty classification of middle ear reconstructions with AMEI and this is shown in Table 2 .

Active Middle Ear Implant Systems

VSB (MED-EL™)

The VSB is an electromagnetic device manufactured by Vibrant MED EL (MED EL Corporation, Innsbruck, Austria). It has been on the market since 1996 and is the most widely studied and most commonly implanted AMEI worldwide.

The VSB is shown in Figure 1 and comprises an external part, the audio processor (AP), and an implanted part, the Vibrating Ossicular Prosthesis (VORP). The AP is worn on the head and con-

Table 2. Classification of middle ear reconstructions with AMEI (Vibroplasty) – adapted from Beleites et al. [3]

Vibroplasty	Description	Subtype	Coupling location	AMEI
Type A	Intact chain	A1	TM, malleus handle	–
		A2	Incus body, malleus head	VSB, Carina
		A3	Incus long process	VSB, Carina
		A4	Stapes footplate	VSB, Carina
Type B	Interrupted/reconstructed chain	B1	Incus body	VSB, Carina
		B2	LP incus, stapes head	Esteem, VSB, Carina
Type C	Membrane coupling inner ear	C1	Round window	Esteem, VSB, Carina
		C2	Oval window/footplate	VSB, Carina
		C3	Third window	–
Type D	Inner ear fluids coupling	D1	Through round window	–
		D2	Through oval window	VSB
		D3	Through third window	–

TM, tympanic membrane; LP, long process.

tains the microphones, the digital signal processing unit and a zinc-air battery as the power source. The implantable aspect of the VSB consists of a receiver coil, a conductor link and a floating mass transducer (FMT).

The device was developed for patients with SNHL who are not able to wear CHA. Originally, the FMT was connected to the long process of the incus after mastoidectomy and posterior tympanotomy with a wide facial recess approach. The FMT was positioned parallel to the stapes to induce movements along the axis of the stapes. Several years after its "classic" introduction, Coletti et al. [4] described the placement of the FMT against the round window membrane in 2006. Since then, other alternative placements have been introduced and couplers that couple the FMT to various parts of the ossicular chain and cochlear windows developed. These adaptations have made the VSB not only suitable for patients with SNHL with an intact ossicular chain but also for patients with CHL or MHL, for example, following cholesteatoma surgery or in cases with congenital aural atresia. The current range of couplers are demonstrated in Figure 1 and are utilized to connect the FMT to the short or long process of the incus, to the stapes or to the round window membrane. Busch et al. [5] showed that the performance with different coupling modalities were equally good in patients with mild to moderate hearing loss.

The risk of directly coupling the FMT to the ossicular chain or cochlear windows is the potential for an iatrogenic conductive or SNHL. In a systematic review of hearing preservation following VSB surgery for SNHL, Bruchhage et al. [6] reported that most studies demonstrated an insignificant alteration in pre- to postoperative audiometry between 500 and 6,000 Hz of between 1 and 3 dB HL. In studies reporting adverse events following VSB surgery, the most common or serious complications were aural fullness (27%), taste disturbances (9%), revision surgery (7%) and facial nerve palsy (1%). Implant failure rates fell from the first generation to the second generation VSB from 14 to 2.6%.

Bruchhage et al. [6] in their study also made a comparison of the hearing benefit of incus vibroplasty for SNHL compared to CHA between the frequency range of 500 and 4,000 Hz. They re-

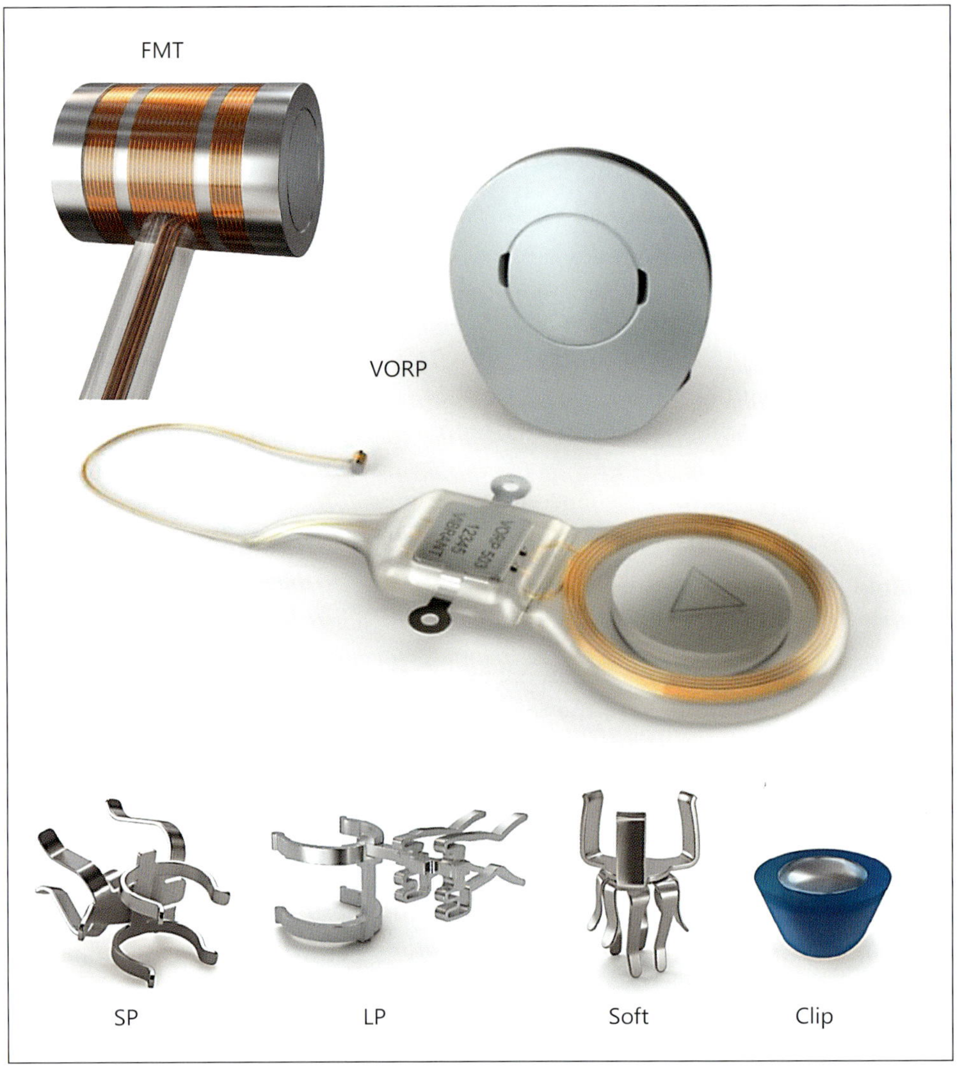

Fig. 1. Vibrant Soundbridge (MED EL) and couplers. FMT, floating mass transducer; VORP, vibrant ossicular prosthesis; SP, short process of the incus coupler; LP, long process of the incus coupler; soft, soft coupler to the round window; clip, clip coupler to stapes head. Courtesy of MED-EL corporation.

ported that in 6 studies of 108 patients, the functional gain was significantly better with the VSB, with a gain from 12.9 to 33.4 dB HL for the VSB and 7.5 to 27 dB HL for hearing aids. It is, however, debatable whether a proper comparison was made in 6 out of these 7 studies by using functional gain and comparing linear devices to a compression technique device like the VSB (see previous remarks). In the study by Saliba et al. [7], the functional gain of the VSB was less than that of the CHA. This was the most valuable study based on the fact that it compared gain and speech perception of the VSB to a CHA in the contralateral ear. Both devices shared the same Signia processor and therefore had bilateral similar processing. Significantly better scores were found with the CHA; on average, the gain was 10 dB higher with the CHA than with the VSB. We, therefore, recommend to only use the VSB in patients with SNHL below 65 dB HL ($PTA_{0.5-2\,kHz}$) as proposed by Verhaegen et al. [8] in cases where a CHA cannot be applied.

Vibroplasty in the presence of an interrupted, malformed or absent ossicular chain provides an important alternative in hearing rehabilitation for individuals with chronic middle ear disease and a clinical contraindication for CHA. These patients have often had multiple surgical procedures where ossiculoplasty has failed to improve hearing or the resultant anatomy has made the use of hearing aids difficult. Round window vibroplasty has been demonstrated to be safe, in most cases stable, and effective [9]. An analysis by Skarzynski et al. [10] showed that in their 3-year follow-up of 21 patients with round window vibroplasty, 2 cases had to undergo revision surgery (10%). Several studies [11–13] have also shown that a lot of attention needs to be paid to adequate coupling of the FMT against the round window membrane. This is more easily achieved by using the recently introduced couplers.

The reported functional gain of the VSB using vibroplasty techniques for mixed/ CHL is reported to range from 13 to 60 dB HL [3, 14–17]. The wide variation probably reflects the inappropriate use of functional gain in MHL or conductive HL. In a systematic review by Ernst et al. [17], it was shown that the functional gain was stable over a 3-year period. Mojallal et al. [18] found better hearing performance in patients who had round window vibroplasty than in those with a bone conduction device in both quiet and competing background noise. In particular, the round window VSB was found to be a better option for the treatment of MHL than a bone conduction device if preoperative bone conduction thresholds were between 35 and 50 dB HL. A systematic review conducted by the Australian MSAC evaluated the safety and effectiveness of AMEI compared to BAHA and demonstrated that the MEI is at least as safe as the BAHA, with the latter having significantly more wound complications [19]. Again, it must be kept in mind that the functional gain is influenced by the width of the air-bone gap and does not completely reflect the performance. In addition, new more powerful BCDs (Ponto 3 SuperPower by Oticon Medical and the BAHA® 5 SuperPower by Cochlear™) have been introduced in the market and the difference in effective gain between AMEI and these BCDs probably is smaller but needs further investigation. Patients with CHL or MHL can be served adequately by VSB vibroplasty when coupling is effective and when preoperative bone conduction thresholds are <50 dB HL. The latter is crucial to maintain a proper dynamic hearing range of 35 dB HL [2, 20, 21].

Studies have demonstrated a high patient satisfaction with the VSB applied for both SNHL and CHL/MHL when compared to conventional hearing aids. Subjective satisfaction is demonstrated in the quality of life visual analog scales, abbreviated profile of hearing aid benefit questionnaires and on the Glasgow benefit inventory when compared to conventional hearing aids [6, 17, 22, 23]. These results must be interpreted in the knowledge that most patients receiving a VSB are likely to have already tried and failed with a CHA for a range of reasons.

There are some limited studies investigating the cost effectiveness of the VSB. These have demonstrated a range of cost per QALY of AMEI implantation. Snik et al. [24] reported a cost of EUR 18,655 per QALY for the use of the VSB in SNHL in patients with severe otitis external. Edfeldt et al. [23] reported a cost per QALY of EUR 7,259 for VSB in SNHL, compared to EUR 12,502 when used in CHL and MHL. Health interventions with a cost-utility ratio of less than GBP 23,000/QALY (EUR 26,920/QALY) are typically considered cost-effective in the United Kingdom [25], which has one of the stringent

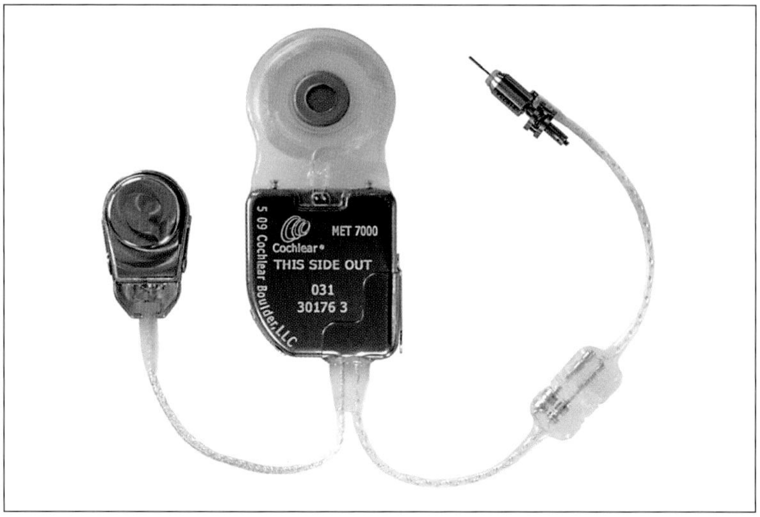

Fig. 2. Carina® (Cochlear Limited). Courtesy of Cochlear Limited.

criteria for cost effectiveness. VSB compares favorably to BAHA which has an estimated cost of EUR 16,085/QALY. The figures reported by the authors were accurate at the time the papers went to press (between 2006 and 2013) but do not take into account inflation, changes in the costs of implants and surgery or other fiscal influences.

Carina® Device (Cochlear)

The Cochlear™ Carina® Middle Ear Implant System (previously the Otologics FIMOS (Fully Implantable Ossicular Stimulator) is a fully implantable AMEI that electromechanically drives the ossicular chain through an actuator with a probe that is placed against the short process of the incus. Previously, the probe was placed in a hole that was created by KTP laser. This is no longer necessary and intraoperative measurements that assist in adequate placement and loading of the probe against the intact ossicular chain. It received a CE mark in 2006 for SNHL and in 2007 for MHL. The device has undergone significant developments since its introduction and these have been necessary to address the initial high device failure rates. Debeaupte et al. [26] reported the device survival rates at 2 years of 0, 76.1, 84.2, 81.8, and 100% for 5 of the successive generations of the Carina. The increasing reliability with the Cochlear Carina was confirmed in a study by Lefebvre et al. [27].

The device (Fig. 2) includes a subcutaneous microphone and a battery that is charged transcutaneous, taking approximately 45 min. Each charge lasts approximately 32 h. A remote control is used to turn the device on and off and controls the volume. The manufacturer reports that the battery life of the Carina is at least 10 years with usage of 16 h per day, although there is no published literature to support this longevity. The Carina can also be used with an external Button™ AP and this extends the range of amplification in both SNHL and CHL/MHL.

The implanted microphone is typically placed on the mastoid; it collects sound and sends it to the processor. The signal is then amplified, processed and sent to the actuator. The actuator is mounted on a bracket that guides its trajectory to the body of the incus. The bracket is connected with self-tapping screws to the cortical bone of the mastoid. The mastoidectomy can be limited in size if access is only required to the body of the incus. Depending on the type of hearing loss and anatomy of the ear, different coupling sites can be

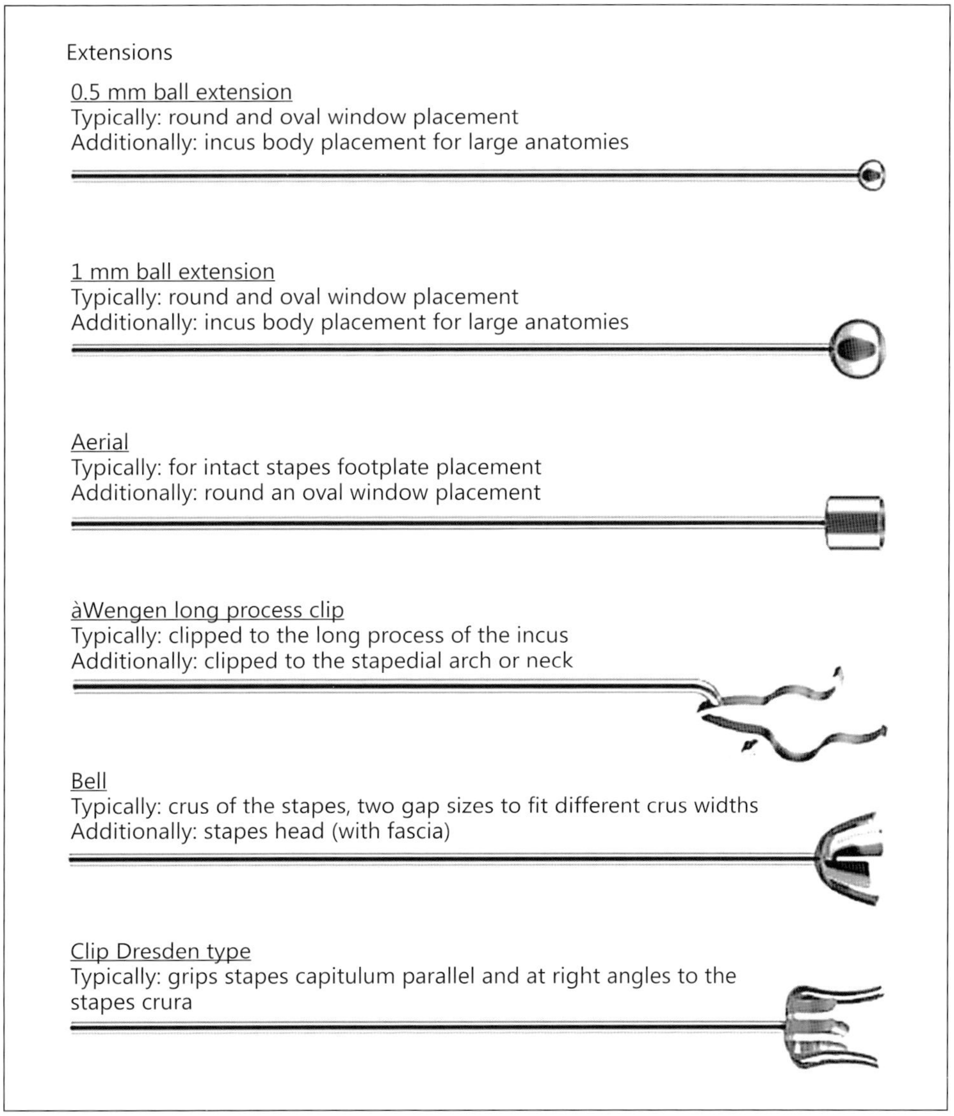

Fig. 3. Actuator extensions for Carina.

used to transfer the energy to the cochlea. For this purpose, several actuator extensions have been introduced to connect the actuator to different parts of the ossicular chain remnants (Fig. 3). The BELL and CliP Dresden type extensions can be used to connect the actuator to the stapes, the AERIAL can be used to connect the actuator to the stapes footplate and the 1.0 and 0.5 mm Ball extensions can be used to connect the actuator to the round or oval window. The LP Clip àWengen can also be used to connect the actuator to the long process of the incus. The correct coupling load of the transducer is evaluated using a device called the transducer loading assistant.

The acoustic performance and quality of sound perception of a fully implantable AMEI is dependent on the implanted microphone. With an internal microphone, there is the risk of undesired somatosounds and feedback. The Carina's microphone contains 2 microphones housed within a single unit. These microphones are antagonistic, with the external microphone capturing environmental sounds and the internal microphone capturing somatosounds. The microphone placement is in the mastoid area with variations in the method used, including placement in a subcutaneous pocket between the skin and the sternocleidomastoid muscle near the mastoid tip or fixing it over the mastoid surface close to the mastoid tip [28]. It is advised that patients be informed that some somatosounds may be perceived after implantation with the Carina, particularly when moving the head towards the implant side. The manufacturer reports that the adaptation period is 6 months when the microphone is attached to the skull and 8–10 months when it is placed in a soft tissue pocket in the neck region. Feedback can be a potential problem with the internal microphone. Carina system feedback is typically reported as a high-pitched "squealing" tone [27]. In cases where the feedback issues cannot be overcome, it may be necessary to resort to the button microphone.

Lefebvre et al. [27] report on 62 recipients (66 ears) with moderate to severe SNHL. They reported a high satisfaction rate among implanted patients with an average daily use of 15 h per day. At the first fitting, feedback was reported for 37% of recipients reducing to 20% at 1 year. Those with continued feedback reported lower levels of satisfaction. Complications were reported as low with 2 cases of microphone body extrusion and 5 cases of device failure with the historic Otologics Carina T1 device. Fifteen of the 66 ears were implanted with the post 2014 Cochlear Carina with no failures at 2 years.

Uhler et al. [29] reported on 58 patients implanted with the Otologics Carina at 11 different US sites as part of the phase IIB FDA clinical trial. Postoperative unaided air conduction thresholds worsened from baseline to activation, but at 12 months no changes were >10 dB. Aided results revealed no change in functional gain or performance on word recognition scores when compared to an appropriately fitted CHA. Subjective satisfaction ratings on the abbreviated profile of hearing aid benefit revealed a significant early improvement at 3 months, but this was reduced at 12 months. At 1-year conclusion of the trial, 13 of 58 subjects (22%) in the overall study had been explanted [29].

Bruschini et al. [28], in a series of 26 patients (32 implants) for both SNHL and CHL/MHL, reported <2 dB HL change between pre- and postoperative air conduction thresholds. They reported a 9% explant rate (1 failure, 1 infection, 1 chronic feedback) and a 12.5% re-operation rate (1 to move microphone, 2 to cover exposed cables and 1 loss of contact of actuator). Martin et al. [30] reported on 11 patients with a prior stapedioplasty or tympanoplasty who had a Carina implant on the RW. Two years after the operation system was activated, an average functional gain of 29 ± 5 dB HL was observed in 8 of 11 patients. There were 2 postoperative infections (18%) requiring device removal and resulting in a "dead ear" in one patient. There was 1 device failure (9%). In a small study by Savas et al. [31], where 9 patients with both SNHL and CHL/MHL were implanted, no statistically significant differences were found between CHA and the Carina implant with regard to hearing amplification and speech discrimination. They did, however, find improved patient satisfaction on the Glasgow Benefit Inventory.

ESTEEM (Envoy Medical)

The Esteem® Hearing Implant (Envoy Medical Corporation, USA) is used to rehabilitate SNHL. It is a totally implantable device and has been available in Europe since 2006 and in the USA since 2010. The device is indicated for adult patients with bilateral, moderate to severe SNHL, good speech discrimination (mean aided free-

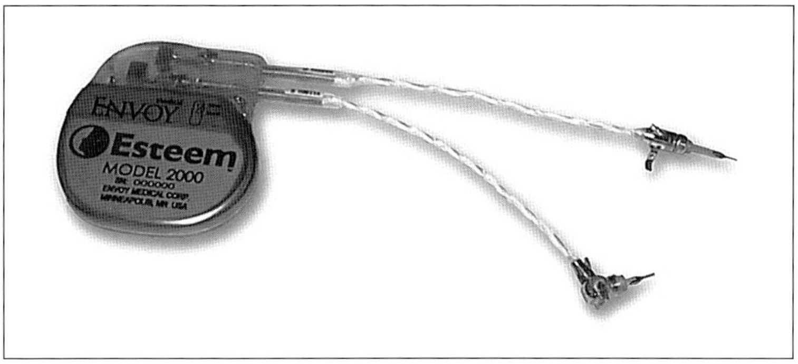

Fig. 4. Esteem® (Envoy Medical). Courtesy of Envoy Medical.

field speech discrimination >50%) [32] and normal middle ears, who have a medical contraindication for a CHA or choose not to wear them. Typically, the ear with the poorest functional hearing is selected for implantation.

The implant consists of a titanium dual-channel sound processor containing the battery and 2 piezoelectric transducers called the driver and the sensor that extend into the middle ear (Fig. 4). The device is microphone free, with the sensor being coupled to the body of the incus to detect tympanic membrane motion. A normal, patent external auditory canal and tympanic membrane are therefore essential. The implant amplifies the signal and transmits this to the head of the stapes via the driver. A tympanomastoidectomy is performed widely, exposing the facial recess to accommodate the driver. The chorda tympani nerve is sacrificed in about 60% of the cases. To prevent feedback, implantation requires separation of the incudostapedial joint and resection of the distal segment of the long process of the incus. Transducers are contained in the mastoid cavity with hydroxyapatite cement, the sensor is coupled to the incus using glass ionomeric cement and the driver is cemented to the stapes. The resultant effect is a maximal conductive hearing on top of the SNHL unless the device is active. In the event of device failure or explantation, this CHL may need to be addressed with an ossiculoplasty.

Some studies have demonstrated that the Esteem device may provide effective bandwidth that exceeds 8 kHz. Low distortion permits increasing acoustic gain (can reach up to +55 dB) without compromising audibility. An open ear canal eliminates the occlusion effect and maintains directionality [32, 33].

The manufacturer states that the battery life of the Esteem depends on device use, with a life range from 4.5 years (24 h per day/7 days per week) to 9 years (8 h per day/7 days per week). However, this may be as short as 2.8 years with continuous exposure to loud noise. The battery can be changed as a surgical procedure under local anesthesia.

Kraus et al. [32] reported on 57 subjects implanted with the Esteem system. Candidates had bilateral, mild to severe SNHL and speech discrimination greater than 40%. They demonstrated good functional gain, good word recognition scores and no postsurgical changes in bone conduction thresholds. In their series, there were 3 revision surgeries for limited benefit (5%), 2 wound infections (one requiring explantation) and one temporary delayed facial paralysis. The majority of subjects considered their device to be equal to or much better than their own CHA. They concluded that hearing results with the Esteem were superior to best-fit hearing aids.

Monini et al. [22] compared the hearing outcomes of 15 adults with an Esteem device to those obtained for CHA. In all the subjects, speech reception thresholds and word recognition scores

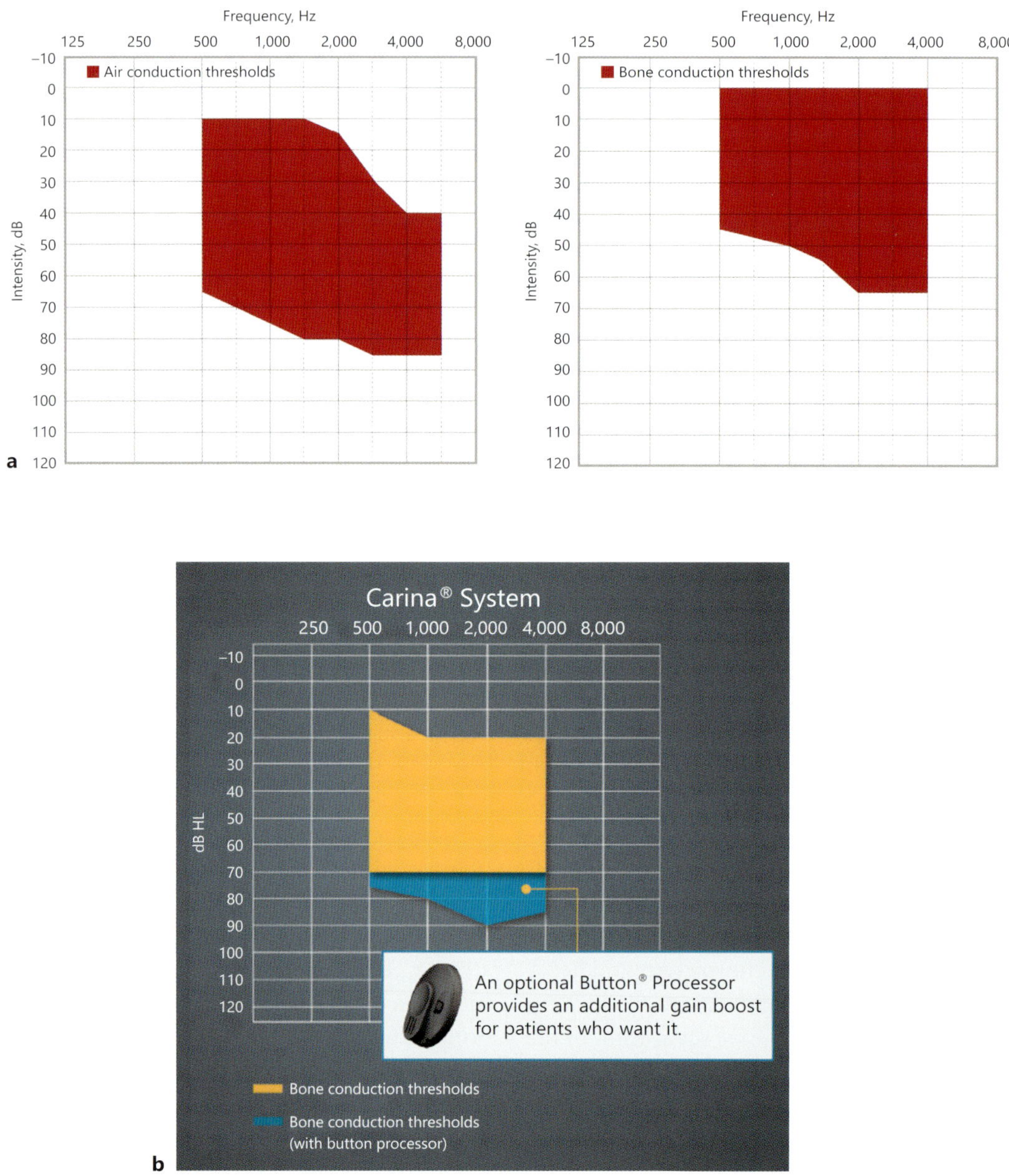

5

(*For figure 5c, d and legend see next page.*)

showed improvement both with CHA and the Esteem with respect to the unaided situation.

Gerard et al. [34] reported on thirteen recipients of the Esteem. In their series, there was high patient satisfaction compared to previous hearing aid use with good functional gain and no autophony. They found that the mean gain was 25 ± 11 dB, with the best results between 500 and 3,000 Hz. However, there were high complication rates, with 2 patients (15%) being explanted

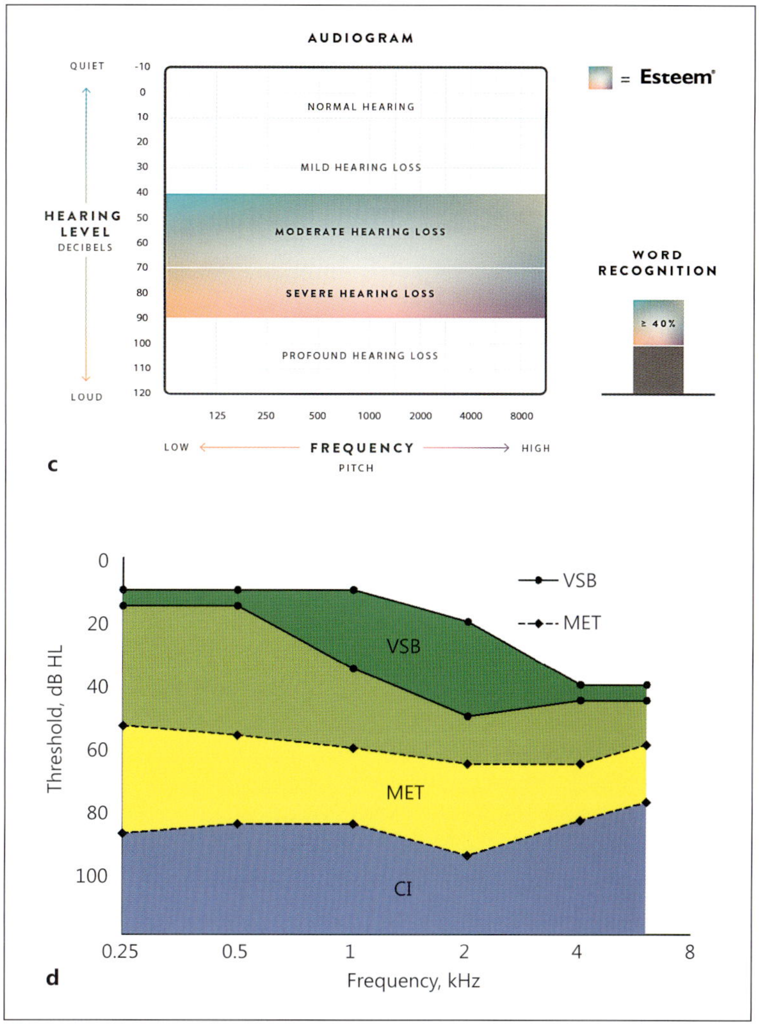

Fig. 5. a–d Audiometric indications of AMEI.

for infection, 3 patients (23%) requiring revision surgery for deteriorating function, disruption of the chorda tympani (61.5%) and one temporary facial palsy.

Audiometric Indications for AMEI

The company recommended audiometric indications for the application of the VSB, Carina and Esteem are demonstrated in Figure 5a–c, respectively. The Cochlear MET, the same device as the Carina but without the implanted microphone, is no longer available, but was shown to provide more amplification than the VSB [7]. The recommended audiometric indications for the VSB and MET in this paper differ from those of the companies: an overview of the applications for the VSB, MET and cochlear implants is shown in Figure 5d. Maximum thresholds for the Carina will be lower due to feedback but may be similar when the external Button™ AP is used. Further research is necessary to establish the maximum application thresholds for all the devices and to evaluate the performance in patients with CHL or MHL. These results should be compared to those obtained for CHA.

MRI Compatibility

MRI is an important and rapidly expanding area in diagnostic imaging. It is regarded as the standard of care for soft tissue imaging, in particular that of the brain and spinal cord. It is estimated that a majority of individuals will require an MRI scan at some stage during their life and as such it is important when considering AMEI [35].

The principal concerns regarding the use of MRI in the presence of AMEI are:

- Powerful magnetic fields may demagnetize or damage the electrical components in the implants.
- Radiofrequency energy may result in heating that can cause tissue damage.
- The artefact caused by the implant may impair the diagnostic usefulness of the scan.

AMEI can be divided into MRI conditional, posing no hazard in a specified MRI environment with specified conditions of use, and MRI unsafe, posing a hazard in all MRI environments [36, 37].

The current implant of the VSB, the VORP 503, is MRI conditional and can be imaged in closed-bore MRI scanners up to 1.5 Tesla with the AP removed. This is a result of a change in the magnet design used in the FMT and receiver stimulator. These magnet advances are not present in the VORP 502, which is MRI unsafe and should not enter an MRI suite or come in close proximity to other sources of strong magnetic fields. Company literature regarding the Carina state that it is MRI unsafe. The Envoy Esteem relies on a piezoelectric transducer that is made up of piezoelectric crystals that are inert within a magnetic field. In Europe, the Esteem implants are regarded as MRI conditional up to 3 Tesla, provided the device is turned off [38]. Conversely in the USA, the company literature states that recipients are not able to undergo MRI examination or be in close proximity to an MRI scanner as this might result in damage to their device [39].

Conclusion

Previous systematic reviews have concluded that while a majority of studies are of moderate or poor quality, data support the safety and gain from AMEI that is comparable with CHA up to certain levels of hearing loss [2, 40]. Above these levels, CHA provide more gain than AMEI and if there is a clinical contraindication for CHA, cochlear implantation with hearing preservation surgery should be considered as the long-term alternative.

The literature clearly demonstrates a role for hearing rehabilitation in patients who for a variety of reasons are not able to utilize CHA. The VSB is the most widely reported AMEI with good safety and reliability data, and with an established application range. The Carina, based on previous measurements of the MET device, is probably a more powerful device than the VSB, however, the feedback of the implantable microphone poses limits to the gain it provides. The big disadvantage of the Esteem device is that the long process of the incus needs to be removed, which means that when the processor is not worn, an additional air-bone gap is introduced. It is clear to see the potential patient advantage of having a fully implantable hearing aid as they are able to use it all the time, during all activities and it does not attract the social stigma of a CHA. However, there remain concerns regarding the effective gain, device reliability, microphone and battery duration. Further research on the Carina and Esteem devices is essential to establish the application criteria and to obtain long-term reliability data as is already available for the VSB.

Acknowledgments

Professor Ad Snik is acknowledged for his valuable and critical comments on this paper.

Disclosure Statement

The authors declare no conflict of interest.

References

1 Dillon H: Hearing Aids; ed 1. New York, Thieme Verlag, 2001.
2 Snik A: Auditory Implants. http://www.snikimplants.nl.
3 Beleites T, Neudert M, Bornitz M, Zahnert T: Sound transfer of active middle ear implants. Otolaryngol Clin North Am 2014;47:859–891.
4 Colletti V, Soli SD, Carner M, Colletti L: Treatment of mixed hearing losses via implantation of a vibratory transducer on the round window. Int J Audiol 2006; 45:600–608.
5 Busch S, Lenarz T, Maier H: Comparison of alternative coupling methods of the vibrant soundbridge floating mass transducer. Audiol Neurotol 2016;21: 347–355.
6 Bruchhage KL, Leichtle A, Schönweiler R, et al: Systematic review to evaluate the safety, efficacy and economical outcomes of the Vibrant Soundbridge for the treatment of sensorineural hearing loss. Eur Arch Otorhinolaryngol 2017; 274:1797–1806.
7 Saliba I, Calmels M-N, Wanna G, et al: Binaurality in middle ear implant recipients using contralateral digital hearing AIDS. Otol Neurotol 2005;26:680–685.
8 Verhaegen VJ, Mylanus EA, Cremers CW, Snik AF: Audiological application criteria for implantable hearing aid devices: a clinical experience at the Nijmegen ORL clinic. Laryngoscope 2008;118: 1645–1649.
9 Colletti L, Mandala M, Colletti V: Long-term outcome of round window Vibrant SoundBridge implantation in extensive ossicular chain defects. Otolaryngol Head Neck Surg 2013;149:134–141.
10 Skarzynski H, Olszewski L, Skarzynski PH, et al: Direct round window stimulation with the Med-El Vibrant Soundbridge: 5 years of experience using a technique without interposed fascia. Eur Arch OtoRhinoLaryngology 2014;271: 477–482.
11 Pennings RJ, Ho A, Brown J, van Wijhe RG, Bance M: Analysis of vibrant soundbridge placement against the round window membrane in a human cadaveric temporal bone model. Otol Neurotol 2010;31:998–1003.
12 Arnold A, Stieger C, Candreia C, Pfiffner F, Kompis M: Factors improving the vibration transfer of the floating mass transducer at the round window. Otol Neurotol 2010;31:122–128.
13 Gostian AO, Pazen D, Ortmann M, et al: Impact of coupling techniques of an active middle ear device to the round window membrane for the backward stimulation of the cochlea. Otol Neurotol 2015;36:111–117.
14 Luers JC, Huttenbrink KB: Vibrant soundbridge rehabilitation of conductive and mixed hearing loss. Otolaryngol Clin North Am 2014;47:915–926.
15 Verhaegen VJ, Mulder JJ, Cremers CW, Snik AF: Application of active middle ear implants in patients with severe mixed hearing loss. Otol Neurotol 2012; 33:297–301.
16 Verhaert N, Desloovere C, Wouters J: Acoustic hearing implants for mixed hearing loss: a systematic review. Otol Neurotol 2013;34:1201–1209.
17 Ernst A, Todt I, Wagner J: Safety and effectiveness of the Vibrant Soundbridge in treating conductive and mixed hearing loss: a systematic review. Laryngoscope 2016;126:1451–1457.
18 Mojallal H, Schwab B, Hinze A-L, Giere T, Lenarz T: Retrospective audiological analysis of bone conduction versus round window vibratory stimulation in patients with mixed hearing loss. Int J Audiol 2015;54:391–400.
19 1137 – Middle Ear Implant for Sensorineural, Conductive and Mixed Hearing Losses Description of Medical Service. www.msac.gov.au/internet/msac/publishing.nsf/Content/1137-public.
20 Zwartenkot JW, Snik AF, Mylanus EA, Mulder JJ: Amplification options for patients with mixed hearing loss. Otol Neurotol 2014;35:221–226.
21 Reinfeldt S, Taghavi H, Eeg-Olofsson M, Hakansson B: New developments in bone-conduction hearing implants: a review. Med Devices Evid Res 2015;8:79.
22 Monini S, Bianchi A, Talamonti R, Atturo F, Filippi C, Barbara M: Patient satisfaction after auditory implant surgery: ten-year experience from a single implanting unit center. Acta Otolaryngol 2017;137:389–397.
23 Edfeldt L, Stromback K, Grendin J, et al: Evaluation of cost-utility in middle ear implantation in the "Nordic School:" a multicenter study in Sweden and Norway. Acta Otolaryngol 2014;134:19–25.
24 Snik AF, van Duijnhoven NT, Mylanus EA, Cremers CW: Estimated cost-effectiveness of active middle-ear implantation in hearing-impaired patients with severe external otitis. Arch Otolaryngol Head Neck Surg 2006;132:1210–1215.
25 Shiroiwa T, Sung YK, Fukuda T, Lang HC, Bae SC, Tsutani K: International survey on willingness-to-pay (WTP) for one additional QALY gained: what is the threshold of cost effectiveness? Health Econ 2010;19:422–437.
26 Debeaupte M, Decullier E, Tringali S, et al: Evolution of the reliability of the fully implantable middle ear transducer over successive generations. Otol Neurotol 2015;36:625–630.
27 Lefebvre PP, Gisbert J, Cuda D, Tringali S, Deveze A: A retrospective multicentre cohort review of patient characteristics and surgical aspects versus the long-term outcomes for recipients of a fully implantable active middle ear implant. Audiol Neurotol 2016;21:333–345.
28 Bruschini L, Berrettini S, Forli F, Murri A, Cuda D: The Carina© middle ear implant: surgical and functional outcomes. Eur Arch Otorhinolaryngology 2016; 273:3631–3640.
29 Uhler K, Anderson MC, Jenkins HA: Long-term outcome data in patients following one year's use of a fully implantable active middle ear implant. Audiol Neurotol 2016;21:105–112.

30 Martin C, Deveze A, Richard C, et al: European results with totally implantable carina placed on the round window: 2-year follow-up. Otol Neurotol 2009;30: 1196–1203.
31 Savaş VA, Gündüz B, Karamert R, et al: Comparison of Carina active middle-ear implant with conventional hearing aids for mixed hearing loss. J Laryngol Otol 2016;130:340–343.
32 Kraus EM, Shohet JA, Catalano PJ: Envoy esteem totally implantable hearing system: phase 2 trial, 1-year hearing results. Otolaryngol Head Neck Surg 2011;145:100–109.
33 Shohet JA, Kraus EM, Catalano PJ: Profound high-frequency sensorineural hearing loss treatment with a totally implantable hearing system. Otol Neurotol 2011;32:1428–1431.
34 Gerard JM, Thill MP, Chantrain G, Gersdorff M, Deggouj N: Esteem 2 middle ear implant: our experience. Audiol Neurootol 2012;17:267–274.
35 Ferreira AM, Costa F, Tralhão A, Marques H, Cardim N, Adragão P: MRI-conditional pacemakers: current perspectives. Med Devices (Auckl) 2014;7: 115–124.
36 Azadarmaki R, Tubbs R, Chen DA, Shellock FG: MRI Information for Commonly Used Otologic Implants. Otolaryngol Neck Surg 2014;150:512–519.
37 Schnabl J, Wolf-Magele A, Pok SM, Hirtler L, Heinz G, Sprinzl GM: Magnetic resonance imaging compatibility of a new generation of active middle ear implant: a clinically relevant temporal bone laboratory study. Otol Neurotol 2016;37:e222–e227.
38 http://envoymedical.de/MRI.
39 Invisible Hearing™ Taking the Next Step. https://www.fda.gov/downloads/Adviso...andThroatDevicesPanel/UCM194364.pdf.
40 Tysome JR, Moorthy R, Lee A, Jiang D, O'Connor AF: Systematic review of middle ear implants: do they improve hearing as much as conventional hearing AIDS? Otol Neurotol 2010;31:1369–1375.

Neil P. Donnelly
Department of Otolaryngology
Cambridge University Hospitals NHS Foundation Trust
Box 48, Hills Road
Cambridge CB2 0QQ (UK)
E-Mail neil.donnelly@addenbrookes.nhs.uk

Lloyd SKW, Donnelly NP (eds): Advances in Hearing Rehabilitation.
Adv Otorhinolaryngol. Basel, Karger, 2018, vol 81, pp 57–65 (DOI: 10.1159/000485586)

Brain Plasticity and Rehabilitation with a Cochlear Implant

Colette M. McKay

The Bionics Institute of Australia and, Department of Medical Bionics, The University of Melbourne, Melbourne, VIC, Australia

Abstract

The functional changes that occur in the brain due to deafness may affect the way the auditory system processes sound after cochlear implantation. Brain plasticity plays a crucial role in the success of cochlear implantation to facilitate or develop spoken language in profoundly deaf individuals. The functional plasticity that occurs in postlingually deaf adults during periods of deafness can both support and hinder speech understanding with a cochlear implant, depending on the nature and degree of functional changes. Evidence so far suggests that the strategies people use to communicate while deaf may influence whether the functional changes are adaptive or maladaptive. In the case of children with congenital deafness, evidence is very strong for a sensitive period in which auditory input must be restored if subsequent oral language is to be developed successfully. Successful oral language use and speech understanding in individuals implanted after 7 years of age depends strongly on the pre-implant use of hearing aids and auditory-verbal communication. Future research should focus on how to harness our growing knowledge of brain plasticity to optimize the outcomes of cochlear implantation in each individual.

Introduction

This chapter describes how the functional changes that occur in the brain due to deafness may affect the way the auditory system processes sound after cochlear implantation. Two separate populations of cochlear implant (CI) users are the focus of this chapter: adults who have been implanted after suffering a postlingual deafness and children or adults who are congenitally deaf. In adults with postlingual deafness, the auditory system has developed normally, but undergoes changes after the person acquires deafness, probably due to the decaying of phonological memory and the increased reliance on visual communication. In children who are congenitally deaf, the lack of early auditory input can lead to a delayed or abnormal development of the cortical structures and networks that support higher auditory function, such as oral language development. In both these populations, the abnormal function of the central auditory system is possibly a major factor underlying the unexplained variability in benefit that CI users gain from the CI. For example, Lazard et al. [1] found that only around 10% of variability in speech understanding in adult CI users could be accounted for by factors, such as duration of deafness and duration of implant use. Similarly, Niparko et al. [2] have shown that, although age at implantation has a large impact on outcomes for children, even those who are implanted at the earliest age acquire oral language skills on average at half the rate of normal hearing children, with rates varying between that of normal hearing children and virtually no language development.

In both children and adults, whether pre- or postlingually deaf, the factors that lead to poor speech understanding or language acquisition after cochlear implantation are complex, including peripheral and central physiological factors and environmental factors, and these different types of factors possibly interact with each other. Recent research using imaging and electrophysiological techniques has shown that the processing of sensory stimuli in the brain of deaf individuals differs from that of people with normal hearing. Furthermore, some of these differences are correlated with the ability to understand speech after implantation. Such plastic changes are induced by auditory deprivation.

Information about brain plasticity comes from imaging studies. Before implantation, all of the main imaging methods have been used in research studies: functional magnetic resonance imaging (fMRI), positron emission tomography (PET) and electroencephalography (EEG). Due to the limitations of using fMRI in CI users, studies imaging the brain of CI users have mostly used PET or EEG. Functional near-infrared spectroscopy (fNIRS) has become mature in recent years, and there are recent studies that have used fNIRS to image brain activity in CI users [3–5]. fNIRS has the advantage in this population of being non-invasive and quiet, and is not affected by electrical artefact as is EEG. It has greatly improved the spatial resolution over EEG and has better temporal resolution than PET. Advances in these imaging techniques provide an opportunity to develop rehabilitation or habilitation strategies that are individually optimized based on objective measures of brain function.

From animal studies, we know that congenital deafness can lead to deficient development of cortical structures. For example, Kral et al. [6] have argued that auditory deprivation through congenital deafness essentially leads to a loss of connectivity between the primary auditory cortex and other areas of the auditory system and widespread brain deficits in processing information beyond the auditory cortex. Similarly, Fallon et al. [7] have described how the auditory cortex is changed by the reintroduction of auditory input after prolonged periods of congenital deafness in guinea pigs. Although there is a wealth of physiological data from animal studies that have researched the effects of deafness and the re-introduction of hearing on the central auditory system, the main focus of this chapter will be the research that has been undertaken with human cochlear implant users that relates to speech understanding and language acquisition. In particular, the chapter focuses on work that is relevant to the successful recovery or development of speech understanding after cochlear implantation. The chapter is divided into 2 main sections: the first discusses adults with postlingual deafness and the second discusses children and adults with congenital deafness.

Adults with Postlingual Deafness

Deafness versus Normal Hearing

Generally, in postlingually deaf adults, speech understanding increases after implantation rapidly in the first 3 months and reaches an asymptote at around 12 months after implantation. Successful rehabilitation depends both on the extent of adaptive or maladaptive plasticity that has occurred before implantation and the extent to which the brain can reclaim or optimize auditory processing networks after implantation. Some studies described below have taken a cross-sectional approach and compare the brain activity of experienced CI users to that of normal hearing listeners. In this case, the differences seen are the net result of these 2 types of plasticity. Other studies have imaged CI users before or shortly after implantation and associated this data with speech understanding after 6–12 months. These studies investigate the influence of plasticity due to auditory deprivation on later speech understanding with the implant. A third type of study follows each CI user longitudinally to determine what changes occur in the brain as an experience with the CI is acquired.

The effect of periods of deafness on brain function in adults who are postlingually deaf has been studied using various imaging techniques. These studies have shown functional differences between deaf people and normal-hearing people in resting state or in response to sensory stimuli. These differences are driven both by the lack of peripheral auditory input into auditory processing areas of the brain, and by the altered communication strategy of the deaf person, with an increased reliance on visual information.

Oral language communication is a multisensory activity, involving integration of auditory, visual and somatosensory senses. Thus, there are multisensory networks in the cortex that support speech understanding. It is not surprising, then, that these networks are altered by the absence of auditory stimulation, either showing increased activation by non-auditory stimuli, or leading to cross-modal plasticity, where areas normally dedicated to auditory processing are altered to process visual or somatosensory information.

Several studies have documented increased visual skills (e.g., motion detection) in hearing impaired people compared to normally hearing people, particularly for stimuli in the peripheral visual field. Many of the early investigations studied congenitally profoundly deaf native signers [8, 9], thus combining the effects of congenital deafness and use of sign language. However, more recent studies have documented improved speech reading skills in postlingually deafened non-signing adults. For example, Rouger et al. [10] evaluated speech reading skills for disyllabic French words in 97 postlingually deaf CI candidates before implantation, immediately after implantation, and 12 months later. Accuracy scores were significantly higher (30–35% mean correct) than for normal-hearing people (9.7% mean correct) and remained unchanged throughout the whole test period. Supra-normal speech reading skills are probably supported by increased efficiency of resources at cortical level that are devoted to visual processing. This functional plasticity due to auditory deprivation may or may not support the adaptation to a re-instated auditory input with a CI. Rouger et al. [10] showed that the newly implanted CI users also showed greater multisensory integration when attending to audio-visual speech stimuli than normal-hearing listeners who were listening to spectrally degraded speech. They suggested that this enhanced integration may support adaptation to a new CI. However, this hypothesis has not been specifically tested.

Lee et al. [11] were one of the first to suggest that deafness may induce cross-modal plasticity in adults. They used PET to compare resting-state metabolism in 9 profoundly deaf adults and 9 age-matched normal-hearing listeners. They found that glucose metabolism in some auditory areas was lower than in normally hearing people, but significantly increased with duration of deafness. They proposed that, during periods of deafness, the auditory areas begin to contribute resources to non-auditory processing and thus become active again in spite of the lack of peripheral auditory input. Many subsequent imaging studies have more directly demonstrated that visually presented information is processed in deaf people in areas of the brain normally dedicated to processing auditory information. A recent study reported by Dewey and Hartley [12], for example, supported this cross-modal plasticity hypothesis. They used fNIRS to show that the auditory cortex in adult deaf CI candidates was activated by simple visual stimuli (a reversing checker board) to a greater degree than in normal-hearing listeners. Rouger et al. [13] also showed that the temporal voice-sensitive area (located in the anterior regions of the superior temporal cortex in the right hemisphere) is abnormally activated by a visual speech reading task in newly implanted CI users, but the activity decreases as the auditory speech understanding recovers. They proposed that this cross-modal reorganization, which re-allocates cortical resources from auditory to visual speech processing in this cortical area, may aid the audio-visual integration of speech after implantation.

Plastic changes to networks involved in phonological processing have also been observed in postlingually deaf adults. For example, Lazard et al. [14], using fMRI, compared activity evoked by speech and non-speech imageries in the left and right posterior superior temporal gyrus/supramarginal gyrus (PSTG/SMG). These areas are normally specialized for phonological processing in the left hemisphere and environmental sound processing in the right hemisphere. Their results suggested the abnormal recruitment of the right PSTG/SMG region for phonological processing in deaf individuals, and they hypothesized that this represented a maladaptive plasticity.

Predicting Cochlear Implant Outcomes

As can be seen from the discussion above, there are differing hypotheses about whether functional plasticity that occurs during periods of deafness is adaptive or maladaptive for auditory processing recovery after cochlear implantation. Two studies that measured evoked potentials to simple visual stimuli in experienced CI users [15, 16] suggested that CI users with poor speech understanding had visual responses that were less focused on the visual cortex, and had greater activation in the auditory area than those with good speech understanding. Both research groups deduced or suggested that gross cross-modal plasticity was therefore maladaptive for CI outcomes. However, since the participants were experienced CI users, it is possible to posit different interpretations. For example, all the CI users may have exhibited similar cross-modal plasticity before implantation but only those who did not get benefit from the CI were still maintaining the visual processing in auditory areas after at least a year of implant use.

Studies that use imaging data collected pre-implantation or immediately post-implantation to test whether the data predict later speech understanding (6–12 months after implantation) can throw light on the adaptive or maladaptive nature of plasticity due to auditory deprivation. The results of these studies demonstrate the adaptive or maladaptive influence of the changes that occurred while the person was deaf and the influence of those changes on the speed of adaptation to the implant in the post-implantation year. Lazard et al. [17], using fMRI, studied phonological processing using a visually presented imagined phonological task in which CI candidates were asked to determine whether written words were rhyming or not. Those with good speech understanding outcomes after implantation showed an activation pattern that was consistent with them using the normal phonological pathway to do the task. This pathway connects the auditory cortex to the pre-frontal cortex in a dorsal route via the pre-motor cortex. In contrast, those CI candidates with poor later outcomes activated a ventral pathway (in the temporal cortex) normally associated with a lexical-semantic understanding.

Strelnikov et al. [18], using PET imaging, measured the response to auditory and audio-visual speech and resting state activity in CI users within one month of CI activation and their speech understanding 6 months after CI activation. They found that speech understanding after 6 months was positively correlated with activity in the left inferior frontal cortex, and with activity in the right occipital cortex, but negatively correlated with activity in the right middle superior temporal gyrus/sulcus. CI users with later good recovery of auditory speech understanding had greater activity levels in right visual cortex and less activity in the right middle superior temporal gyrus/sulcus than those with poor recovery. The authors deduced that recovery of auditory speech understanding is supported by intra-modal compensation in the visual area (perhaps evoked by enhanced focus on lip-reading during periods of deafness) and less cross-modal reorganization in the auditory superior temporal gyrus/sulcus. The authors noted that activity in the right temporal area was identified both in their study, as negatively correlated with later speech understanding, and by Rouger et al. [13], as having greater activity in CI users than normal-hearing listeners, but decreasing over time after implantation. They suggested therefore that auditory recovery must depend on the reversibility of the cross-modal reorganization of this area.

Relevance of Plasticity to Rehabilitation Success
It is evident from the above research that the nature and degree of functional changes that occur due to auditory deprivation can have a large impact on the ability of a person to recover their speech understanding ability after cochlear implantation. It is likely that increased visual skills such as lip-reading and increased multisensory integration can help a person learn to interpret the electrical signal from a CI. However, some changes are likely to be maladaptive: for example, the increased use of the right hemisphere and ventral processing pathways in the left hemisphere to understand speech. Lazard et al. [19] suggested that those people who relied more on written communication rather than lip-reading while deaf were more likely to experience maladaptive plasticity that limits their success with the cochlear implant. The time is now right for research to address 2 important questions. First, "What simple clinical test could be used to provide better prognostic information to adults before implantation?" Second, "With knowledge of an individual's plastic functional changes to their language networks, is it possible to devise individual hearing therapies that aim to reverse maladaptive changes?" The further development of fNIRS as a user-friendly clinical tool may facilitate this important research.

Congenital Deafness

Early Language Development in Infants
In children and adults with congenital deafness, an important factor is the influence of deafness on the early development of language processing pathways in the brain. There is now much evidence, both from human and animal studies, of a sensitive developmental period for establishing the important multisensory networks required to understand oral speech. In this section, we discuss this evidence and its relevance to habilitation of children and adults with congenital deafness.

Much research has demonstrated the impressive ability of normal-hearing new-born infants to process and recognize aspects of spoken language. As the evidence from animal studies makes it clear, early input to the primary auditory cortex is crucial for the development of connections to the auditory association areas and lack of input causes widespread functional connectivity changes throughout the cortex [20, 21]. Sharma et al. [22] have reviewed evidence for developmental sensitive periods, and evidence for cross-modal plasticity in deaf children. The cortical auditory evoked potential (CAEP) can provide a physiological marker for maturation of the auditory cortex in infants [23]. The P1 response, which originates in the auditory cortex and is present at birth, systematically decreases in latency with age [24], and the N1 potential, which originates in the higher order auditory cortex, begins to emerge [25] around the age of 3 years in normal-hearing children. Sharma et al. [24] showed that children implanted under the age of 3.5 years demonstrated maturation of the P1 response after implantation, whereas those implanted after 7 years did not achieve such

language, it is likely to tap into the usual multisensory network that underlies oral speech. Bayazit et al. [37] studied 49 prelingually deaf children who were implanted after the age of 5 years. They found that, over 2 years, a significant number of children who were implanted between 5 and 14 years old shifted from total communication to auditory verbal communication, but not in the group implanted between 15 and 22 years old. They noted that successful auditory verbal communication after implantation was related to consistent hearing aid use from early childhood and use of auditory verbal communication before implantation. Both of the above studies are consistent with the success of the implantation relying on the development of oral language pathways before the sensitive period cut-off of 7 years, either through use of residual hearing and hearing aids, or by familiarity with oral language structure through lip reading and somatosensory information.

Conclusions

Brain plasticity plays a crucial role in the success of a CI to facilitate or develop spoken language for profoundly deaf individuals. The functional plasticity that occurs in postlingually deaf adults during periods of deafness can both support and hinder speech understanding with a CI, depending on the nature and degree of the functional changes. Evidence so far suggests that the strategies people use to communicate while deaf may influence whether the functional changes are adaptive or maladaptive. In the case of children with congenital deafness, evidence is very strong for a sensitive period in which auditory input must be restored if subsequent oral language is to be developed successfully. Successful oral language use and speech understanding in individuals implanted after 7 years of age depends strongly on the pre-implant use of hearing aids and auditory verbal communication. Future research should focus on how to harness our growing knowledge of brain plasticity to optimize the outcomes of cochlear implantation in each individual.

Acknowledgments

The Bionics Institute acknowledges the support it receives from the Victorian Government through its Operational Infrastructure Support Program. The author is supported by a Veski Innovation Fellowship.

References

1 Lazard DS, Vincent C, Venail F, Van de Heyning P, Truy E, Sterkers O, Skarzynski PH, Skarzynski H, Schauwers K, O'Leary S, et al: Pre-, per- and postoperative factors affecting performance of postlinguistically deaf adults using cochlear implants: a new conceptual model over time. PLoS One 2012;7:e48739.

2 Niparko JK, Tobey EA, Thal DJ, Eisenberg LS, Wang NY, Quittner AL, Fink NE: Spoken language development in children following cochlear implantation. JAMA 2010;303:1498–1506.

3 McKay C, Shah A, Seghouane AK, Zhou X, Cross W, Litovsky R: Connectivity in language areas of the brain in cochlear implant users as revealed by fNIRS. Adv Exp Med Biol 2016;894:327–335.

4 Olds C, Pollonini L, Abaya H, Larky J, Loy M, Bortfeld H, Beauchamp MS, Oghalai JS: Cortical activation patterns correlate with speech understanding after cochlear implantation. Ear Hear 2016;37:e160–e172.

5 Sevy AB, Bortfeld H, Huppert TJ, Beauchamp MS, Tonini RE, Oghalai JS: Neuroimaging with near-infrared spectroscopy demonstrates speech-evoked activity in the auditory cortex of deaf children following cochlear implantation. Hear Res 2010;270:39–47.

6 Kral A, Kronenberger WG, Pisoni DB, O'Donoghue GM: Neurocognitive factors in sensory restoration of early deafness: a connectome model. Lancet Neurol 2016;15:610–621.

7 Fallon JB, Shepherd RK, Irvine DR: Effects of chronic cochlear electrical stimulation after an extended period of profound deafness on primary auditory cortex organization in cats. Euro J Neurosci 2014;39:811–820.

8 Neville HJ, Lawson D: Attention to central and peripheral visual space in a movement detection task. III. Separate effects of auditory deprivation and acquisition of a visual language. Brain Res 1987;405:284–294.

9 Brozinsky CJ, Bavelier D: Motion velocity thresholds in deaf signers: changes in lateralization but not in overall sensitivity. Brain Res Cogn Brain Res 2004;21:1–10.

10 Rouger J, Lagleyre S, Fraysse B, Deneve S, Deguine O, Barone P: Evidence that cochlear-implanted deaf patients are better multisensory integrators. Proc Natl Acad Sci U S A 2007;104:7295–7300.
11 Lee JS, Lee DS, Oh SH, Kim CS, Kim JW, Hwang CH, Koo J, Kang E, Chung JK, Lee MC: PET evidence of neuroplasticity in adult auditory cortex of postlingual deafness. J Nucl Med 2003;44:1435–1439.
12 Dewey RS, Hartley DE: Cortical cross-modal plasticity following deafness measured using functional near-infrared spectroscopy. Hear Res 2015;325:55–63.
13 Rouger J, Lagleyre S, Demonet JF, Fraysse B, Deguine O, Barone P: Evolution of crossmodal reorganization of the voice area in cochlear-implanted deaf patients. Hum Brain Mapp 2012;33:1929–1940.
14 Lazard DS, Lee HJ, Truy E, Giraud AL: Bilateral reorganization of posterior temporal cortices in post-lingual deafness and its relation to cochlear implant outcome. Hum Brain Mapp 2013;34:1208–1219.
15 Doucet ME, Bergeron F, Lassonde M, Ferron P, Lepore F: Cross-modal reorganization and speech perception in cochlear implant users. Brain 2006;129:3376–3383.
16 Sandmann P, Dillier N, Eichele T, Meyer M, Kegel A, Pascual-Marqui RD, Marcar VL, Jancke L, Debener S: Visual activation of auditory cortex reflects maladaptive plasticity in cochlear implant users. Brain 2012;135:555–568.
17 Lazard DS, Lee HJ, Gaebler M, Kell CA, Truy E, Giraud AL: Phonological processing in post-lingual deafness and cochlear implant outcome. Neuroimage 2010;49:3443–3451.
18 Strelnikov K, Rouger J, Demonet JF, Lagleyre S, Fraysse B, Deguine O, Barone P: Visual activity predicts auditory recovery from deafness after adult cochlear implantation. Brain 2013;136:3682–3695.
19 Lazard DS, Innes-Brown H, Barone P: Adaptation of the communicative brain to post-lingual deafness. Evidence from functional imaging. Hear Res 2014;307:136–143.
20 Kral A, Eggermont JJ: What's to lose and what's to learn: development under auditory deprivation, cochlear implants and limits of cortical plasticity. Brain Res Rev 2007;56:259–269.
21 Kral A, Tillein J, Heid S, Klinke R, Hartmann R: Cochlear implants: cortical plasticity in congenital deprivation. Prog Brain Res 2006;157:283–313.
22 Sharma A, Campbell J, Cardon G: Developmental and cross-modal plasticity in deafness: evidence from the P1 and N1 event related potentials in cochlear implanted children. Int J Psychophysiol 2015;95:135–144.
23 Wunderlich JL, Cone-Wesson BK: Maturation of CAEP in infants and children: a review. Hear Res 2006;212:212–223.
24 Sharma A, Dorman M, Spahr AJ: A sensitive period for the development of the central auditory system in children with cochlear implants: implications for age of implantation. Ear Hear 2002;23:532–539.
25 Sussman E, Steinschneider M, Gumenyuk V, Grushko J, Lawson K: The maturation of human evoked brain potentials to sounds presented at different stimulus rates. Hear Res 2008;236:61–79.
26 Yoshinaga-Itano C, Sedey AL, Coulter DK, Mehl AL: Language of early- and later-identified children with hearing loss. Pediatrics 1998;102:1161–1171.
27 Lee HJ, Giraud AL, Kang E, Oh SH, Kang H, Kim CS, Lee DS: Cortical activity at rest predicts cochlear implantation outcome. Cereb Cortex 2007;17:909–917.
28 Humphries T, Kushalnagar P, Mathur G, Napoli DJ, Padden C, Rathmann C, Smith S: Bilingualism: A pearl to overcome certain perils of cochlear implants. J Med Speech Lang Pathol 2014;21:107–125.
29 Campbell R, MacSweeney M, Woll B: Cochlear implantation (CI) for prelingual deafness: the relevance of studies of brain organization and the role of first language acquisition in considering outcome success. Front Hum Neurosci 2014;8:834.
30 Lyness CR, Woll B, Campbell R, Cardin V: How does visual language affect crossmodal plasticity and cochlear implant success? Neurosci Biobehav Rev 2013;37:2621–2630.
31 Wie OB, Falkenberg ES, Tvete O, Tomblin B: Children with a cochlear implant: characteristics and determinants of speech recognition, speech-recognition growth rate, and speech production. Int J Audiol 2007;46:232–243.
32 Geers A, Brenner C, Nicholas J, Uchanski R, Tye-Murray N, Tobey E: Rehabilitation factors contributing to implant benefit in children. Ann Otol Rhinol Laryngol Suppl 2002;189:127–130.
33 Altvater-Mackensen N, Grossmann T: The role of left inferior frontal cortex during audiovisual speech perception in infants. Neuroimage 2016;133:14–20.
34 Altvater-Mackensen N, Mani N, Grossmann T: Audiovisual speech perception in infancy: the influence of vowel identity and infants' productive abilities on sensitivity to (mis)matches between auditory and visual speech cues. Devel Psychol 2016;52:191–204.
35 Kos MI, Deriaz M, Guyot JP, Pelizzone M: What can be expected from a late cochlear implantation? Int J Ped Otorhinolaryngol 2009;73:189–193.
36 Ling D, Clarke BR: Cued speech: an evaluative study. Am Ann Deaf 1975;120:480–488.
37 Bayazit YA, Altinyay S, Cevizci R: Delayed prelingual cochlear implantation in childhood and puberty. Int J Ped Otorhinolaryngol 2015;79:146–150.

Colette M. McKay
Bionics Institute
384–388 Albert St
East Melbourne VIC 3002 (Australia)
E-Mail cmckay@bionicsinstitute.org

Lloyd SKW, Donnelly NP (eds): Advances in Hearing Rehabilitation.
Adv Otorhinolaryngol. Basel, Karger, 2018, vol 81, pp 66–73 (DOI: 10.1159/000485544)

Hearing Preservation Cochlear Implant Surgery

Iain A. Bruce[a] · Ingo Todt[b]

[a]Royal Manchester Children's Hospital, Manchester, UK; [b]Klinikum Bielefeld, Department of Otolaryngology, Head and Neck Surgery, Bielefeld, Germany

Abstract

Cochlear implantation (CI), with attempted preservation of residual natural low-frequency hearing, is an increasingly accepted application of this technology, with potential benefits to the patient when listening in noise and in music appreciation. The full extent of the benefits of combining preserved natural hearing and electrical stimulation remain under evaluation. Various factors appear to influence the success of hearing preservation (HP) during CI, including electrode design, surgical approach, insertional trauma, steroid usage and patient factors. Currently, combining or contrasting outcomes of CI with attempted HP is difficult due to the use of heterogeneous outcome measures. Until we have a full understanding of the benefits of preserving residual low-frequency hearing during CI, there is merit in attempting to preserve all residual hearing. Likewise, preserving residual low-frequency hearing is a useful surrogate marker for atraumatic electrode design and insertion.

Introduction

The insertion of a cochlear implant electrode array into the cochlea with the collateral intention of preserving residual natural hearing, represents one of the most significant recent advances in cochlear implantation (CI). Preserving low-frequency hearing enables the patient to potentially benefit from acoustic stimulation of low frequencies and electrical stimulation of higher frequencies (sometimes referred to as electroacoustic stimulation [EAS]) [1]. This potential to combine electrical and natural hearing continues to drive evolution in the design and application of CI, with the potential that increasing numbers of patients can potentially benefit from this technology.

Candidacy

When considering candidacy for CI with attempted hearing preservation (HP), it is important to consider the nature of the therapeutic intent, which is influenced by the degree of residual natural hearing. CI with HP is usually performed on patients who meet the criteria for CI at mid- and high-frequencies, but have variable degrees of residual low-frequency hearing. Three broad groups of patients are considered for CI with HP, as defined by the amount of residual low-frequency hearing and the possibility of benefiting from a combined CI and conventional hearing aid (HA) device: (i) low-frequency hearing in the normal range, (ii) low-frequency hearing considered to be readily amplified using a combined CI and HA device (e.g., MED-EL Duet 2 audio processor or Cochlear Nucleus Hybrid System), (iii) low-frequency hearing likely to be insufficient to benefit from using a combined CI and HA. The hearing threshold below which the patient is considered to be unlikely to benefit from a combined CI and HA device is not fully determined, with certain manufacturers recommending a "cut-off" of 65 dB HL at 125, 250 and 500 Hz [2, 3]. Further improvements in HA technology and greater understanding of the benefits of combined acoustic and "electrical" hearing will refine the recommendations available to clinicians.

HP Rates

No standardized methodology exists for reporting the outcome of CI with attempted preservation of residual hearing, and published success rates vary widely [1, 4]. The resulting difficulty in comparing results between studies in a meaningful manner is further compounded by variability in the study populations reported. Most studies use postoperative pure tone audiometric thresholds to determine success, with there being a paucity of evidence regarding patient-reported benefit. A classification system has been suggested by Skarzynski et al. [5] that calculates the % preservation relative to the degree of preoperative residual hearing. The % preservation (S) is then classified as "complete" (75–100%), "partial" (25–75%), "minimal" (1–25%) or "loss of hearing" (no detectable hearing). Likewise, there is no standardized time point after CI when the level of preservation of residual natural hearing should be measured. This is important to consider as evidence exists for subsequent deterioration in preserved hearing over time [4, 6]. A study of 13 adults [6] following CI with HP reported 43% "complete," 50% "partial" and 7% "minimal" preservation at initial postoperative testing using the Skarzynski et al. [5] HP classification system, which dropped to 25% "complete," 12.5% "partial" and 37.5% "minimal" preservation at 2 years, using the MED-EL Flex EAS electrode. However, patients obtained benefit in speech discrimination and quality of life regardless of whether initially preserved natural hearing was preserved into the medium term.

Although the majority of case series have concentrated on CI with HP in adults, there is some evidence for the success of CI with HP in children and young people, with the suggestion that better HP is achieved in the pediatric population [1]. One study using MED-EL Flex portfolio electrode arrays has reported successful HP in 13/14 young people at an average follow-up of 2 years 10 months, using the presence of measurable hearing thresholds to determine success (Bruce et al. [4]). In this cohort, 50% complete preservation of hearing (difference between the preoperative and postoperative masked bone conduction thresholds at low frequencies [125–500 Hz] less than 10 dB) was achieved and the rest maintained hearing to within 40 dB at 6 weeks. Three patients did, however, have a delayed profound hearing deterioration. Another study in 5 children ranging from 13 months to 14 years of age has reported complete preservation using MED-EL Flex EAS electrodes [7]. A 90% rate of at least partial HP (loss <40 dB HL on pure tone average at 250, 500 and 1,000 Hz) has been reported in a study of 31 children, ranging in age from 1 to 19 years [8]. Using the Skarzynski et al. [9] HP classification system to evaluate the Cochlear Nucleus Slim Straight electrode (Nucleus CI422), 15/19 children (6–18 years) have been demonstrated to have had "partial" or "complete" HP at initial activation, subsequently stable when tested at 24 months postoperatively [9].

There is currently limited evidence regarding the effect of revision CI surgery on natural hearing preserved after initial CI surgery, with evidence from some centers reporting successful replacement of the electrode array without loss of previously preserved natural hearing [2, 4]. There are limited reports suggesting that residual natural hearing can be potentially improved following introduction of an electrode array into the cochlea, postulated as possibly resulting from beneficial changes in basilar membrane mechanics (stiffness) correcting a pre-existing conductive problem [3, 10].

Surgical Technique

The use of an atraumatic electrode array and a refined surgical technique are considered to be of critical importance in achieving HP. With reference to surgical technique, influencing factors can be further divided into: (1) pre-insertional factors, (2) insertional factors and (3) post-insertional factors. Categorizing the importance of these individual factors is currently difficult due to the paucity of available prospective data and limitations of study designs employed.

Pre-Insertional Factors

Pre-insertional factors influencing HP are considered to be important [11]. Preservation of residual hearing has been demonstrated most commonly using the posterior tympanotomy approach to the middle ear, but variations in access route (e.g., suprameatal approach) have also been shown to facilitate HP [12].

Performing a posterior tympanotomy provides wide access to the middle ear, and allows for variation of the insertional angle [13] and proper visualization of the round window, or the promontory for a cochleostomy. Care must be taken during posterior tympanotomy to avoid inadvertent trauma to the ossicular chain, with resultant trauma to the inner ear [14]. Entry of blood into the cochlea has been experimentally shown to have negative effects on the degree of HP [15], emphasizing the importance of meticulous hemostasis. Some authors recommend rinsing the middle ear with antibiotic solution or saline before electrode insertion, with the intention of reducing the risk of infectious contamination of the inner ear during electrode insertion [16]. Steroids are widely used in HP surgery [17], but there is a lack of definitive evidence regarding the ideal mode of delivery (e.g., topical to the middle ear and/or systemic), type of steroid (e.g., triamcinolone, dexamethasone) and dosage. Indeed, whilst Braun et al. [18] have found a positive effect on HP, others have not seen a significant benefit from steroid usage [19]. Steroid-eluting electrodes have provisionally shown positive effects in animal studies [20–22]. Whether the positive steroid effect is directly related to the steroid itself or a fluid-related decrease in the round window opening pressure and the hydrostatic effect remains under discussion [23].

Promontorial lip reduction or cochleostomy drilling should be limited in terms of burr speed to prevent noise trauma [24]. Two factors are important when considering opening of either the round window membrane or endosteum following cochleostomy: (1) atraumacity to limit changes in intra-cochlear pressure and (2) adequate sealing around the electrode at the entry point into the cochlea after implantation. Different tools to open the round window membrane have been shown experimentally to cause significantly different intra-cochlear pressure changes [25]. A diode laser-based opening method has been shown to cause small pressure changes, while a CO_2 laser resulted in high pressure amplitudes. Lower intra-cochlear pressure changes have also been demonstrated experimentally when mechanically opening the round window membrane in wet (transfluid) rather than dry conditions [26], which is in line with clinical observations [27].

Additionally, larger round window opening has been shown experimentally to significantly decrease the intra-cochlear pressure by allowing the fluid to pass out of the cochlea [28]. This is in contradiction to the often performed puncture of the round window to allow the electrode to pass into the cochlea. In vivo studies support the positive effect of a wide round window opening [23]. A disadvantage might be the sealing of the opening after electrode insertion.

Intra-cochlear access has been most commonly reported via the round window approach in the HP literature, but comparably successful HP has been described using a cochleostomy approach, suggesting that the site of access into the cochlea is not a critical factor [3, 29].

Insertional Factors

Speed of advancement of the electrode array into the cochlea appears to be important in HP. Experimentally, it has been shown that increases in intra-cochlear pressure during implantation correlates with the speed of electrode array insertion [30]. Clinical data support this effect by demonstrating a direct correlation between speed of insertion, HP and vestibular effects [31].

The electrode acts as a direct transmitter of manual electrode movements into the inner ear by fast- and slow-hydrostatic pressure changes. These movements are extensively affected even by pre- and post-insertional factors. Different factors influence the stabilization of the electrode during the insertion. There are both external and internal stabilization factors that are important during insertion of the electrode array. One external factor is hand and elbow stabilization to minimize tremor effects [32]. Another uses the walls of the posterior tympanotomy and the superior bony edge of the round window niche to stabilize the electrode as it is inserted. This can be assisted using specific insertion tools [33]. Some types of electrode are internally stabilized as they are inserted through support offered by the walls of the cochlea [34], and this correlates with insertional depth. In which degree the electrode volume design contributes to this effect is a matter of further observation.

Post-Insertional Factors

The effect of post-insertional factors on HP can be underestimated. Experimentally, the effectiveness of the seal around the electrode array at its entry point into the cochlea can be influenced by cochleostomy size, electrode array dimensions and the substance used [35, 36]. Recently, it was shown that resealing can solve a proportion of vestibular problems (Karimi et al., 2016, unpublished) by closing a silent perilymphatic fistula. Ineffective sealing could be responsible for both early and delayed onset perilymph leak with subsequent sensorineural hearing loss, but can also cause conductive hearing loss if the sealing material interferes with the ossicular chain or if there is a subsequent scar formation from the electrode entry point to the stapes [37]. Kiefer et al. [38] described the technique of a punched fascia to deal with this problem. However, even the sealing technique has an effect on intracochlear pressure (Luger et al., 2016, unpublished); a seal with multiple overlaying strips (most surgeons use fascia) causes the lowest pressure changes. Pushing the strips between electrode and cochleostomy/round window edge should be avoided. Since movement of the electrode within the cochlea is translated into pressure changes, the electrode is essentially acting as a loudspeaker [39, 40], uncontrolled contacts with the electrode as well as movements should be limited after the insertion of the electrode since they are directly transmitted into the cochlea as a pressure change. Experiments have suggested that the post-insertional stabilization of the electrode array in the posterior tympanotomy may be important to limit intra-cochlear displacement of the electrode array, which may occur if the electrode is simply stored in the mastoid cavity (Todt et al., 2016e, unpublished). Different techniques for the stabilization of the electrode inside the posterior tympanotomy, such as clips [41, 42], sutures [43], grooves for electrode wings or a bone plate with fibrin glue or a fascia have been described [44]. An adequate pre-storage fixation prevents not only uncontrolled pressure peaks of up to 170 dB, but even a postoperative migration of the electrode.

Implant Choice

The physical characteristics of the implanted electrode are regarded as being a central factor in determining the success of preserving residual natural hearing during CI. As with other factors influencing successful HP, our understanding continues to evolve. There exists consensus that minimizing the intra-cochlear trauma is a critical factor when attempting to preserve residual hearing during CI. As such, it is accepted that the electrode should not be too rigid. The concept of minimizing trauma led to the development of a generation of short electrode arrays designed to avoid contact with the apical region of the cochlea, where residual hearing function remained. With advances in the design of these shorter electrodes and surgical technique, some degree of residual hearing can be consistently preserved [45]. However, evidence now exists that residual hearing can be preserved using a full insertion of a longer length electrode array [1, 3, 4, 46–50]. A study has described successful HP in 12/14 CIs (arbitrarily determined), using a deep insertion of a standard length electrode array, thereby covering the region of residual hearing in the cochlear [3]. If residual hearing can be consistently preserved to an acceptable extent using longer electrodes contacting the more apical regions of the cochlea, then "smart programming" with subsequent stepwise activation of electrodes to match any subsequent hearing loss may prove beneficial to the patient [3, 8, 49]. This may be of particular importance to children and younger adults, where some functionally significant deterioration in residual natural hearing can be expected with aging. It also provides the ability to stimulate the entire cochlea if HP fails. It has been suggested that children are at a higher risk of progressive hearing loss than adults, as their physiology and etiology of hearing loss may make them more susceptible to hearing deterioration and they face more years of potential hearing loss [8, 51]. Further work is needed to determine the exact role of shorter and longer electrode arrays in HP surgery. Perhaps shorter electrode arrays may be advocated when low-frequency hearing is normal or stable over a prolonged period, or the anticipated risk of significant deterioration is low over the predicted lifespan of the patient. Electrode volume may also be important in HP as larger volume electrodes have been shown to result in increased intra-cochlear in fast and hydrostatic pressure changes [30, 52].

Currently, the majority of HP electrodes evaluated in published studies are of a straight design, as opposed to pre-curved. Although, initial experience with pre-curved electrodes demonstrated a higher chance of translocation into the scala vestibuli, evaluation of a novel mid-scala pre-curved electrode (Advanced Bionics HiFocus Mid-Scala) has shown that HP is possible. Using the Skarzynski et al. [5] HP classification system, 53% (17/32 adult ears) had "complete" or "partial" HP at initial activation [53].

Matching the physical characteristics of the electrode array to the morphology of the cochlea may ultimately prove to be the critical factor influencing the choice of electrode array. Work is ongoing to identify methods based on radiological imaging, to quantify the implantable dimensions of the cochlea, but subsequent benefit from this "bespoke" approach to electrode selection has yet to be proved [54]. A recent meta-analysis has not shown any particular electrode design to incur an advantage [1].

Benefits of EAS

Outcomes of EAS

Comparing preoperative HA with postoperative EAS performance, Lorens et al. [55] measured an increase of 40% in monosyllabic word understanding in quiet using an EAS audio processor, when compared with "HA only." Similar results were reported by Gstoettner et al. [56], with a significant improvement in monosyllable recognition in quiet from 9% with "HA only" to 48 and 65% in the "CI-only" and EAS conditions, respectively. Differences for CI and EAS conditions in monosyllable word recognition in noise (10 dB SNR: 56.1% [CI only] and 72.4% [EAS]; 0 dB SNR: 18.6% [CI only] and 33.9% [EAS]) were significant [55]. Additionally, a time-dependent learning effect could be observed with mean monosyllable scores of 78% after 8 months of training with an EAS system [57]. Combined electroacoustic audio processors have been demonstrated to provide benefit in the recognition of musical instruments when compared to conventional CI users [58, 59]. Brockmeier et al. [60] evaluated the music reception abilities of electroacoustic audio processor users and found pitch discrimination to be close to normal hearing performance, but observed persistent problems with rhythm perception and instrument differentiation.

An important factor for the audiological outcome of an EAS/Hybrid system is the degree of residual hearing [61]. Moreover, some adaptation time is necessary before patients are able to reach their optimal performance with an EAS processor [62].

A small number of studies have reported outcome in children fitted with electroacoustic audio processors [47, 63, 64]. In 25 children (mean age at CI 9.5 years, range 4.2–16.6 years), monosyllable recognition scores in quiet increased from 31% preoperatively ("HA only") to 60% in the EAS condition. In noise (+10 dB SNR), a mean increase from 1% preoperatively ("HA only") to 19% in the EAS condition was recorded. Scholz et al. [65] describe inferior results for a group of younger children (2.2 years at CI). They found that 4/6 cases used their electroacoustic audio processor but there was no significant increase in speech understanding when using the EAS device compared to the "CI only" (Oldenburger sentence test [adaptive] in noise S0N90 CI only –4.7 dB vs. hybrid –6.1 dB). Their results may have been affected by the short follow-up period of 8 weeks.

It should also be noted that, in selected cases, speech recognition can be further improved if ipsilateral EAS is combined with an additional contralateral HA [55, 66], although the benefits may be limited. For example, Lenarz et al. [67] described an average improvement of 1.8 dB by adding an HA to the contralateral ear.

Currently, evaluation of the benefit of bilateral EAS is limited. Moteki et al. [68] described 2 patients with bilateral electroacoustic audio processors, in whom a remarkable increase in localization ability and speech understanding in quiet and noise, was demonstrated.

Conclusion

Whilst our understanding of the benefits of preserving residual natural hearing and factors influencing successful preservation during CI continues to evolve, much clinical and basic science research remains to be undertaken. Future advances in this area may include: (1) genetic analysis to predetermine likely initial and long-term success of CI with HP [69], (2) biotechnology-assisted CI (drug-based [e.g., steroid], gene-based [e.g., gene transfection] and cell-based [human stem cells] therapies), and (3) robotic CI to further limit the invasiveness, intracochlear trauma and operator error inherent in the conventional manual procedure.

References

1 Santa Maria PL, et al: Hearing preservation surgery for cochlear implantation: a meta-analysis. Otol Neurotol 2014; 35:e256–e269.

2 Helbig S, et al: Scalar localization by computed tomography of cochlear implant electrode carriers designed for deep insertion. Otol Neurotol 2012;33: 745–750.

3 Bruce IA, et al: Hearing preservation via a cochleostomy approach and deep insertion of a standard length cochlear implant electrode. Otol Neurotol 2011; 32:1444–1447.

4 Bruce IA, et al: Hearing preservation cochlear implantation in adolescents. Otol Neurotol 2014;35:1552–1559.

5 Skarzynski H, et al: Towards a consensus on a hearing preservation classification system. Acta Otolaryngol Suppl 2013;564:3–13.

6 Santa Maria PL, et al: Hearing preservation surgery for cochlear implantation – hearing and quality of life after 2 years. Otol Neurotol 2013;34:526–531.

7 Kuthubutheen J, et al: A case series of paediatric hearing preservation cochlear implantation: a new treatment modality for children with drug-induced or congenital partial deafness. Audiol Neurootol 2012;17:321–330.

8 Brown RF, et al: Residual hearing preservation after pediatric cochlear implantation. Otol Neurotol 2010;31:1221–1226.

9 Skarzynski H, et al: Preservation of cochlear structures and hearing when using the Nucleus Slim Straight (CI422) electrode in children. J Laryngol Otol 2016;130:332–339.

10 Kiefer J, et al: Representation of acoustic signals in the human cochlea in presence of a cochlear implant electrode. Hear Res 2006;221:36–43.

11 von Ilberg C, et al: Electric-acoustic stimulation of the auditory system. New technology for severe hearing loss. ORL J Otorhinolaryngol Relat Spec 1999;61: 334–340.

12 Postelmans JT, et al: Comparison of two cochlear implantation techniques and their effects on the preservation of residual hearing. Is the surgical approach of any importance? Eur Arch Otorhinolaryngol 2014;271:997–1005.

13 Causon A, Verschuur C, Newman TA: A retrospective analysis of the contribution of reported factors in cochlear implantation on hearing preservation outcomes. Otol Neurotol 2015;36: 1137–1145.

14 Jiang D, et al: Equivalent noise level generated by drilling onto the ossicular chain as measured by laser Doppler vibrometry: a temporal bone study. Laryngoscope 2007;117:1040–1045.

15 Radeloff A, et al: Impact of intrascalar blood on hearing. Laryngoscope 2007; 117:58–62.

16 von Ilberg CA, et al: Electric-acoustic stimulation of the auditory system: a review of the first decade. Audiol Neurootol 2011;16(suppl 2):1–30.

17 Rajan GP, et al: The role of preoperative, intratympanic glucocorticoids for hearing preservation in cochlear implantation: a prospective clinical study. Laryngoscope 2012;122:190–195.

18 Braun S, et al: Protection of inner ear function after cochlear implantation: compound action potential measurements after local application of glucocorticoids in the guinea pig cochlea. ORL J Otorhinolaryngol Relat Spec 2011; 73:219–228.

19 Honeder C, et al: Effects of intraoperatively applied glucocorticoid hydrogels on residual hearing and foreign body reaction in a guinea pig model of cochlear implantation. Acta Otolaryngol 2015; 135:313–319.

20 Stathopoulos D, et al: Development of a safe dexamethasone-eluting electrode array for cochlear implantation. Cochlear Implants Int 2014;15:254–263.

21 Farhadi M, et al: Dexamethasone eluting cochlear implant: Histological study in animal model. Cochlear Implants Int 2013;14:45–50.

22 Liu Y, et al: Effects of a dexamethasone-releasing implant on cochleae: a functional, morphological and pharmacokinetic study. Hear Res 2015;327:89–101.

23 Todt I, Mittmann P, Ernst A: Hearing preservation with a midscalar electrode comparison of a regular and steroid/pressure optimized surgical approach in patients with residual hearing. Otol Neurotol 2016;37:e349–e352.

24 Pau HW, et al: Noise exposure of the inner ear during drilling a cochleostomy for cochlear implantation. Laryngoscope 2007;117:535–540.

25 Mittmann P, Ernst A, Todt I: Intracochlear pressure changes due to round window opening: a model experiment. Scientific World Journal 2014;2014: 341075.

26 Mittmann P, et al: Optimisation of the round window opening in cochlear implant surgery in wet and dry conditions: impact on intracochlear pressure changes. Eur Arch Otorhinolaryngol 2016;273: 3609–3613.

27 Anagiotos A, et al: Insertion of cochlear implant electrode array using the underwater technique for preserving residual hearing. Otol Neurotol 2016;37:339–344.

28 Todt I, Ernst A, Mittmann P: Effects of round window opening size and moisturized electrodes on intracochlear pressure related to the insertion of a cochlear implant electrode. Audiol Neurotol Extra 2016;6:1–8.

29 Hassepass F, et al: Radiologic Results and Hearing Preservation With a Straight Narrow Electrode via Round Window Versus Cochleostomy Approach at Initial Activation. Otol Neurotol 2015;36:993–1000.

30 Todt I, Mittmann P, Ernst A: Intracochlear fluid pressure changes related to the insertional speed of a CI electrode. Biomed Res Int 2014;2014:507241.

31 Rajan GP, Kontorinis G, Kuthubutheen J: The effects of insertion speed on inner ear function during cochlear implantation: a comparison study. Audiol Neurootol 2013;18:17–22.

32 Todt I, Ernst A, Mittmann P: Effects of different insertion techniques of a cochlear implant electrode on the intracochlear pressure. Audiol Neurootol 2016; 21:30–37.

33 Todt I, et al: Comparison of the effects of four different cochlear implant electrodes on intra-cochlear pressure in a model. Acta Otolaryngol 2017;137:235–241.

34 Mittmann M, et al: Insertional depth-dependent intracochlear pressure changes in a model of cochlear implantation. Acta Otolaryngol 2017;137:113–118.

35 Robey AB, et al: Effect of cochleostomy size on perilymph fistula control. Laryngoscope 2010;120:373–376.
36 Burghard A, et al: Insertion site and sealing technique affect residual hearing and tissue formation after cochlear implantation. Hear Res 2014;312:21–27.
37 Chole RA, Hullar TE, Potts LG: Conductive component after cochlear implantation in patients with residual hearing conservation. Am J Audiol 2014;23:359–364.
38 Kiefer J, et al: Conservation of low-frequency hearing in cochlear implantation. Acta Otolaryngol 2004;124:272–280.
39 Mueller M, et al: Electro-mechanical stimulation of the cochlea by vibrating cochlear implant electrodes. Otol Neurotol 2015;36:1753–1758.
40 Schraven SP, et al: Vibro-EAS: a proposal for electroacoustic stimulation. Otol Neurotol 2015;36:22–27.
41 Cohen NL, Kuzma J: Titanium clip for cochlear implant electrode fixation. Ann Otol Rhinol Laryngol Suppl 1995;166:402–403.
42 Muller J, Schon F, Helms J: [Reliable fixation of cochlear implant electrode mountings in children and adults – initial experiences with a new titanium clip]. Laryngorhinootologie 1998;77:238–240.
43 Balkany T, Telischi FF: Fixation of the electrode cable during cochlear implantation: the split bridge technique. Laryngoscope 1995;105:217–218.
44 Hüttenbrink KB, et al: Biologic fixation of the electrode cable of cochlea implants. Otorhinolaryngol Nova 2000;10:213–216.
45 Gantz BJ, et al: Preservation of hearing in cochlear implant surgery: advantages of combined electrical and acoustical speech processing. Laryngoscope 2005;115:796–802.
46 Baumgartner WD, et al: Outcomes in adults implanted with the FLEXsoft electrode. Acta Otolaryngol 2007;127:579–586.
47 Skarzynski H, et al: Preservation of residual hearing in children and post-lingually deafened adults after cochlear implantation: an initial study. ORL J Otorhinolaryngol Relat Spec 2002;64:247–253.
48 Punte AK, Vermeire K, Van de Heyning P: Bilateral electric acoustic stimulation: a comparison of partial and deep cochlear electrode insertion. A longitudinal case study. Adv Otorhinolaryngol 2010;67:144–152.
49 Prentiss S, Sykes K, Staecker H: Partial deafness cochlear implantation at the University of Kansas: techniques and outcomes. J Am Acad Audiol 2010;21:197–203.
50 Helbig S, et al: Hearing preservation after complete cochlear coverage in cochlear implantation with the free-fitting FLEXSOFT electrode carrier. Otol Neurotol 2011;32:973–979.
51 Uchanski RM, et al: Two ears and two (or more?) devices: a pediatric case study of bilateral profound hearing loss. Trends Amplif 2009;13:107–123.
52 Mittmann P, et al: Intracochlear pressure changes due to 2 electrode types. Otolaryngol Head Neck Surg 2017;156:712–716.
53 Hunter JB, et al: Hearing preservation outcomes with a mid-scala electrode in cochlear implantation. Otol Neurotol 2016;37:235–240.
54 Alexiades G, Dhanasingh A, Jolly C: Method to estimate the complete and two-turn cochlear duct length. Otol Neurotol 2015;36:904–907.
55 Lorens A, et al: Outcomes of treatment of partial deafness with cochlear implantation: a DUET study. Laryngoscope 2008;118:288–294.
56 Gstoettner W, et al: A new electrode for residual hearing preservation in cochlear implantation: first clinical results. Acta Otolaryngol 2009;129:372–379.
57 Helbig S, Baumann U: Acceptance and fitting of the DUET device – a combined speech processor for electric acoustic stimulation. Adv Otorhinolaryngol 2010;67:81–87.
58 Gfeller KE, et al: Music perception with cochlear implants and residual hearing. Audiol Neurootol 2006;11(suppl 1):12–15.
59 Gfeller K, et al: Accuracy of cochlear implant recipients on pitch perception, melody recognition, and speech reception in noise. Ear Hear 2007;28:412–423.
60 Brockmeier SJ, et al: Music perception in electric acoustic stimulation users as assessed by the Mu.S.I.C. test. Adv Otorhinolaryngol 2010;67:70–80.
61 Gantz BJ, et al: Hybrid 10 clinical trial: preliminary results. Audiol Neurootol 2009;14(suppl 1):32–38.
62 Skarzyński H, et al: Results of partial deafness cochlear implantation using various electrode designs. Audiol Neurootol 2009;14(suppl 1):39–45.
63 Skarzynski H, et al: Partial deafness cochlear implantation in children. Int J Pediatr Otorhinolaryngol 2007;71:1407–1413.
64 Skarzynski H, Lorens A: Electric acoustic stimulation in children. Adv Otorhinolaryngol 2010;67:135–143.
65 Scholz S, Wagner F, Olze H, Todt I, Battmer RD: Benefit of a hybrid speech processor in implanted young children with residual hearing. JSM Health Educ Prim Health Care 2016;2:1028–1031.
66 Baumann U, Helbig S: [Hearing with combined electric acoustic stimulation]. HNO 2009;57:542–550.
67 Lenarz T, et al: Hearing conservation surgery using the hybrid-L electrode. Results from the first clinical trial at the medical university of hannover. Audiol Neurootol 2009;14(suppl 1):22–31.
68 Moteki H, et al: The advantages of sound localization and speech perception of bilateral electric acoustic stimulation. Acta Otolaryngol 2015;135:147–153.
69 Usami S, et al: Patients with CDH23 mutations and the 1555A>G mitochondrial mutation are good candidates for electric acoustic stimulation (EAS). Acta Otolaryngol 2012;132:377–384.

Prof. Iain A. Bruce
Paediatric ENT Department, Royal Manchester Children's Hospital
Manchester University NHS Foundation Trust
Manchester Academic Health Science Centre
Manchester, M13 9WL (UK)
E-Mail Iain.Bruce@cmft.nhs.uk

Lloyd SKW, Donnelly NP (eds): Advances in Hearing Rehabilitation.
Adv Otorhinolaryngol. Basel, Karger, 2018, vol 81, pp 74–80 (DOI: 10.1159/000485546)

Extended Applications for Cochlear Implantation

John Martin Hempel • Florian Simon • Joachim Michael Müller
Department of Otorhinolaryngology, Head and Neck Surgery, Ludwig Maximilians University Munich, Munich, Germany

Abstract
The indications for cochlear implantation (CI) have expanded over the last few years. There is evidence that some adult patients with pre- or perilingual onset of deafness may gain from implantation. Similarly, CI in patients with single-sided deafness may offer significant benefits in terms of quality of life and social as well as academic development. In this setting, directional hearing may be restored and speech comprehension, especially in noise, may be optimized. In patients with intractable tinnitus and profound hearing loss, CI not only improves speech perception, but also helps to reduce the tinnitus in the deaf ear.

Introduction

Cochlear implantation (CI) is one of the most significant achievements in modern medicine. Thanks to the pioneering spirit of innovative and visionary otologists, the indications for cochlear implants are continuously expanding, such that an increasing number of people can benefit from this treatment. The significant benefits of binaural hearing from bilateral cochlear implants (CI) have been demonstrated and form an important milestone in hearing rehabilitation. Today, bilateral CI is considered the gold standard whenever affordable, in children as well as in adults.

Two decades ago, there was still great controversy regarding whether or not CI would provide significant auditory benefit in patients with postlingual single-sided deafness (SSD). Subsequent data have demonstrated that speech comprehension in the deaf ear is improved following CI and that there are benefits in directional hearing and hearing in noise. This has been shown to improve the quality of life. This has demonstrated that the auditory system can effectively integrate electrical hearing with the acoustic hearing of the contralateral ear [1]. The ability of the auditory system to integrate electrical and auditory signals in the same ear has also been demonstrated and has become known as electroacoustic stimulation (EAS). Similarly, CI as a treatment for severe intractable tinnitus is increasingly being offered. Those patients presenting as adults who have been pre- or perilingually deafened are no longer dismissed out of hand as candidates for CI as studies have suggested that some of these people will benefit from the procedure within a limited range of realistic expectations [2, 3]. This article addresses current topics in the extended range of indications for CI.

Single-Sided Deafness

SSD, or unilateral hearing loss, is defined as nonfunctional hearing in one ear, with normal hearing in the other ear. SSD has multiple effects, which often depend on the time when the person became deaf in that ear.

A decade ago, parents of children with SSD were being advised that unilateral hearing loss was unfortunate but did not require any active rehabilitation. It has become apparent, however, that children who have SSD, irrespective of whether the hearing loss is conductive or sensorineural [4], congenital or acquired, are often unable to communicate verbally the hearing difficulties that they experience. Numerous studies have now shown that unilateral hearing loss may have negative effects on speech development, social interaction and academic development [5, 6].

Adults who become suddenly deaf in one ear usually suffer from a loss of binaural hearing, that is, a loss of directional hearing (due to affected interaural timing difference detection, intensity variation and reduced head shadow effect) and a reduction in speech comprehension in noisy environments (because of the reduced head shadow effect, squelch and summation effects through unilateral deafness). In particular, people who are working full time and are also socially active complain of resultant increasing fatigue with loss of concentration and tension in the muscles of the neck and shoulders. Some of these patients become accustomed to the loss of hearing on one side after a certain length of time but others are very frustrated by it. They are also often anxious about relying on one ear and are concerned that they may develop hearing loss in their good ear becoming bilaterally profoundly deaf. These same complaints are vocalized by adolescents and adults who have SSD from childhood. These issues are also particularly important for those patients with partial hearing loss on one side and complete deafness on the other.

With the realization in recent years that unilateral hearing loss should be treated, the technology of contralateral routing of signals (CROS) hearing aids has been improved. These devices allow limited compensation for the unilateral hearing loss in some patients. Similar benefits are achieved with bone conduction hearing aids, but such devices have the great advantage over the CROS hearing aid that the healthy ear does not have to be blocked by an ear mould (occlusion effect), and this leads to greater user acceptance [7]. Both CROS and bone conduction hearing aids are only indirect solutions, however, and the hearing itself is not rehabilitated. They may, in fact, even result in reduced speech comprehension in some hearing situations [8].

Treating SSD with Cochlear Implants

In the treatment of SSD with cochlear implants, we can distinguish three patient groups:

1. Acquired unilateral hearing loss identified early

a. During adulthood, for example, due to idiopathic sudden loss of hearing without further treatment options, a fracture of the petrous bone, a complication of stapes or cholesteatoma surgery, or as a result of the resection of an intralabyrinthine schwannoma

b. During childhood or adolescence, for example, a fracture of the petrous bone or meningitis with unilateral hearing loss

2. Acquired unilateral hearing loss during childhood or adulthood identified late

3. Congenital unilateral hearing loss

a. Identified in childhood, for example, through neonatal hearing screening

b. Identified in adulthood

34 Gordon KA, Wong DD, Papsin BC: Bilateral input protects the cortex from unilaterally-driven reorganization in children who are deaf. Brain 2013; 136(Pt 5):1609–1625.
35 Távora-Vieira D, Boisvert I, McMahon CM, Maric V, Rajan GP: Successful outcomes of cochlear implantation in long-term unilateral deafness: brain plasticity? Neuroreport 2013;24:724–729.
36 Van de Heyning P, Vermeire K, Diebl M, Nopp P, Anderson I, De Ridder D: Incapacitating unilateral tinnitus in single-sided deafness treated by cochlear implantation. Ann Otol Rhinol Laryngol 2008;117:645–652.
37 Mertens G, Kleine Punte A, De Ridder D, Van de Heyning P: Tinnitus in a single-sided deaf ear reduces speech reception in the nontinnitus ear. Otol Neurotol 2013;34:662–666.
38 Távora-Vieira D, Marino R, Acharya A, Rajan GP: The impact of cochlear implantation on speech understanding, subjective hearing performance, and tinnitus perception in patients with unilateral severe to profound hearing loss. Otol Neurotol 2015;36:430–436.
39 Buechner A, Brendel M, Lesinski-Schiedat A, Wenzel G, Frohne-Buechner C, Jaeger B, Lenarz T: Cochlear implantation in unilateral deaf subjects associated with ipsilateral tinnitus. Otol Neurotol 2010;31:1381–1385.
40 Kim DK, Moon IS, Lim HJ, Yoo SY, Heo KW, Bae SC, et al: Prospective, multicenter study on tinnitus changes after cochlear implantation. Audiol Neurootol 2016;21:165–171.
41 Olze H, Knopke S, Gräbel S, Szczepek AJ: Rapid Positive Influence of Cochlear Implantation on the Quality of Life in Adults 70 Years and Older. Audiol Neurootol 2016;21(suppl 1):43–47.
42 Teoh SW, Pisoni DB, Miyamoto RT: Cochlear implantation in adults with prelingual deafness. Part I. Clinical results. Laryngoscope 2004;114:1536–1540.
43 Kumar RS, Mawman D, Sankaran D, Melling C, et al: Cochlear implantation in early deafened, late implanted adults: Do they benefit? Cochlear Implants Int 2016;17(suppl 1):22–25.
44 Schramm D, Fitzpatrick E, Séguin C: Cochlear implantation for adolescents and adults with prelinguistic deafness. Otol Neurotol 2002;23:698–703.
45 Rahne T, Plontke SK: Functional result after cochlear implantation in children and adults with single-sided deafness. Otol Neurotol 2016;37:e332–e340.

PD Dr. med. John Martin Hempel
Department of Otorhinolaryngology, Head and Neck Surgery
Ludwig Maximilians University Munich
Marchioninistrasse 15
DE–81377 Munich (Germany)
E-Mail john-martin.hempel@med.uni-muenchen.de

Lloyd SKW, Donnelly NP (eds): Advances in Hearing Rehabilitation.
Adv Otorhinolaryngol. Basel, Karger, 2018, vol 81, pp 81–92 (DOI: 10.1159/000485542)

Management of Cochlear Nerve Hypoplasia and Aplasia

Simon R. Freeman[a] • Levent Sennaroglu[b]

[a]Department of Otolarygology, Central Manchester University Hospitals NHS Foundation Trust (CMFT), Manchester Academic Health Science Centre (MAHSC), Manchester, UK; [b]Hacettepe University Medical Faculty, Department of Otolaryngology, Ankara, Turkey

Abstract

Approximately 2% of congenital profound deafness cases are due to cochlear nerve (CN) deficiency. MRI is essential to confirm if the nerve is deficient, but because of limitations with resolution, especially when the internal auditory canal is narrowed, it is often unable to distinguish between hypoplasia and aplasia. A full audiometric test battery should always be performed, even if the MRI suggests CN aplasia, as there will sometimes be evidence of audition. Electrically evoked auditory brainstem response testing can be carried out transtympanically via the round window or using an intracochlear test electrode to help determine the status of the CN. If any test suggests the presence of a CN, then cochlear implantation (CI) should be considered. Children should be followed up closely with audiometric, electrophysiological and language assessments to determine the benefits. They may initially show benefit but fail to progress. CI results are variable and often result in poor outcomes with Categories of Auditory Perception scores of <5. Auditory brainstem implantation (ABI) can be considered when CI is contraindicated or fails to provide adequate benefit. This may provide better outcomes, but this form of surgery has greater risks and future device replacement (in case of device failure) may be complicated. Careful patient selection is required when considering ABI as significant learning difficulties make programming extremely challenging. Patients should be given the option of CI first and then ABI. A small minority of patients presenting late (around 2–3 years of age) may be candidates for simultaneous CI and ABI.

Introduction

The terms cochlear nerve (CN) hypoplasia or aplasia describe either a small or absent CN. These malformations have been estimated to occur radiologically in 0.8 and 1.8% of profoundly deaf children [1]. The collective term cochlear nerve deficiency (CND) is commonly used.

Historically, CT scans were used to define cochlear implantation (CI) candidacy. It was recognized that a narrow internal auditory canal (IAC) of less than 2 mm width, known to be associated with CND on temporal bone specimens, often meant a lack of benefit from CI and that this should be considered a contraindication [2, 3]. With the development of MRI, it became possible to directly visualize the vestibulocochlear nerve (VCN) and its branches. Casselman et al. [4] were the first to study MRI findings in children with CND and suggested categorizing it into 2 types. Type 1 consisted of complete aplasia of the VCN; in type 2, the VCN was present (either normal or hypoplastic) but the CN was abnormal (either aplastic or hypoplastic). Type 2 was further subdivided into A (associated with inner ear malformations [IEM]) or B (inner ear normal).

In the decade following the study by Casselman et al. [4], a number of studies were published demonstrating that CI has a role to play in hearing rehabilitation in some of these children, variably using audiometry and electrical stimulation preoperatively to determine candidacy where MRI was equivocal. At the same time, others started to consider the use of auditory brainstem implantation (ABI) in these children [5, 6]. The First Consensus Meeting in 2009 evaluated the early results of ABI in young children and established parameters for use [7]. Four years later, the Second Consensus Meeting considered the entire process including assessment and the longer term results of both CI and ABI in children with CND [8].

This paper presents the current knowledge base related to the management of patients with hypoplastic or aplastic VCN or CN. The utility of MRI as well as audiological and electrophysiological testing in the assessment of these patients will be discussed and the indications for and outcomes of CI and ABI presented.

Preoperative Workup

Radiology

MRI is the only investigation that can evaluate the anatomy of the VCN and its branches and as such is mandatory in the evaluation of congenital profound deafness [4, 9, 10]. Standard sequences of the internal auditory meati (IAM) with T2-weighted gradient echo or turbo spin echo sequences using sub-millimeter slice thicknesses and inter-slice distances provide high resolution with excellent tissue/fluid contrast. Imaging is carried out in the axial plane with bilateral parasagittal images perpendicular to the nerves attained via either multi-planar reconstruction or direct acquisition. The latter gives greater resolution, but at the expense of longer scan times [11]. Scans performed at 3 Tesla provide the best resolution [12]. Young children require sedation as a minimum, while general anesthesia reduces the likelihood of movement artefact. CT is also helpful as this provides better resolution of the bony canals (IAC, cochlear nerve canal [CNC], also known as the cochlear aperture, and facial canal) and identifies the surgical anatomy of the temporal bone. The use of CT alone will miss some cases of CND as this can still occur even when the IAC and CNC are normal [9, 10].

The size, position and variability of the normal 7th and 8th cranial nerves have been studied by a number of authors [4, 13–15]. The normal VCN is visualized leaving the brainstem posterior to the facial nerve (FN). Both nerves traverse the cerebellopontine angle (CPA) in parallel in an anterolateral direction and enter the IAC at the porus acusticus. The diameter of the VCN is usually $1^1/_2$ to 2 times that of the FN (Fig. 1a). The VCN divides into the CN, positioned inferiorly, and the vestibular nerve, positioned superiorly. The latter then divides again to form the superior vestibular nerve and inferior vestibular nerve (Fig. 1b). The points of division and the topographical relationships are variable, but in 90% of cases they divide in the proximal half of the IAC. The CN then passes into the CNC towards the modiolus of the cochlea. The CN in normally hearing ears is approximately 1 mm in diameter with a slightly ovoid shape in cross-section. Its size is similar to the FN, but it may be slightly larger or smaller.

There is little consensus in the literature as to what point an 8th cranial nerve should be considered as hypoplastic. Casselman et al. [4] found

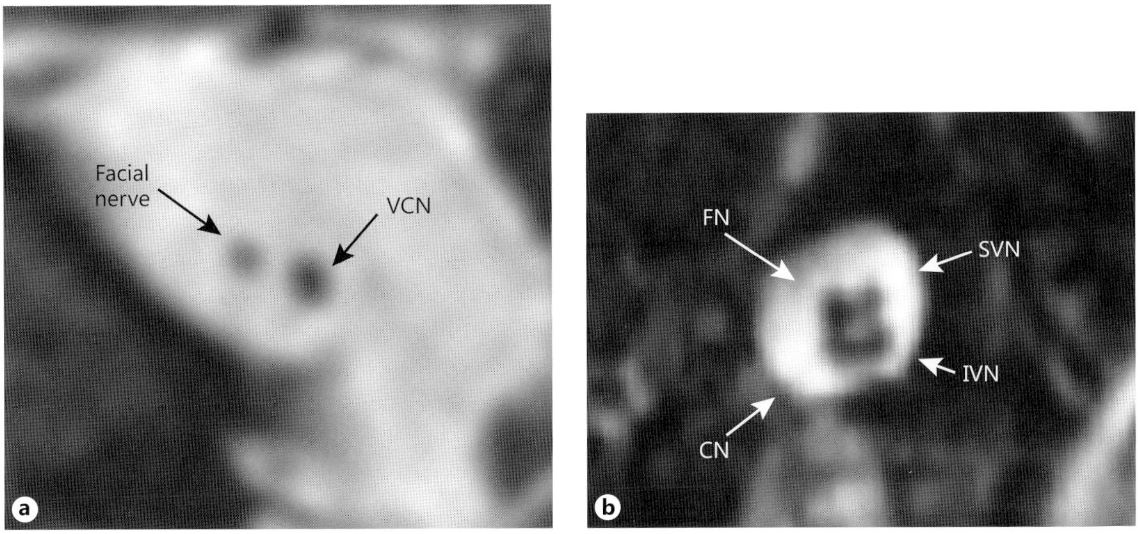

Fig. 1. a T2-weighted high-resolution parasagittal MRI of the cerbellopontine angle demonstrating a normal vestibulocochlear nerve (VCN) and facial nerve. **b** T2-weighted high-resolution parasagittal MRI of the internal auditory meati (IAM) demonstrating a normal cochlear nerve (CN), superior and inferior vestibular nerves (SVN and IVN) and facial nerve (FN).

that the main trunk of the VCN in the CPA was never smaller than the adjacent FN in normally hearing ears and Yamazaki et al. [16] used this cut-off when comparing CI benefit in CND. Most studies have focused only on the more distal CN when trying to determine hypoplasia. Casselman et al. [4] considered the CN to be hypoplastic when it was "much" smaller than the adjacent FN within the IAC. While some authors have used the same definition as Casselman et al. [9, 10, 17], some have more liberally defined hypoplasia as present whenever the CN is smaller than the FN in the mid-portion of the IAC [18–20] and others when it is less than half the diameter of the FN [21]. Clemmens et al. [22] used normative data comparing the relative diameter, area and density between CN and FN and concluded that the CN should be regarded as hypoplastic if the area or diameter were <0.9 of the FN.

Aplasia of the VCN in the CPA is usually apparent on the axial and parasagittal MRI (Fig. 2a, b). Radiological absence of a VCN does not, however, mean that the nerve is not present. This has been clearly demonstrated by Song et al. [23] who reported 2 cases in which hypoplastic VCNs were found during ABI even though none were visualized on MRI. Equally, a CN may not be visualized in the IAC even though a small or rudimentary nerve is present (Fig. 3a, b). There are reports of patients with apparent CN aplasia who clearly demonstrate a small amount of audition or benefit with CI [19, 24]. This has led Birman et al. [19] to suggest classifying CND as per the number of nerves seen in the IAC. It is also important to consider the position of the FN within the temporal bone, which can lie in several different positions in relation to CND and IEMs including an early exit of the IAM, a separate anterior facial canal, traversing the petrous apex or traversing Meckel's cave alongside the trigeminal nerve [25, 26]. If only a single nerve is seen entering the IAM, it is important to exclude an aberrant FN as it could be the VCN [27].

There are a number of reasons why a VCN or CN may not be seen. First, artifacts may occur,

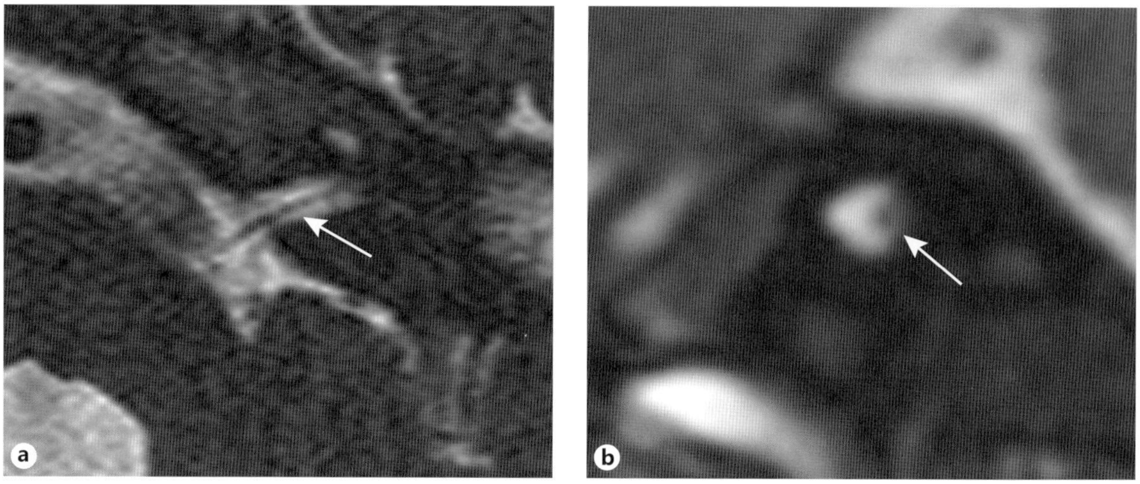

Fig. 2. a T2-weighted high-resolution axial MRI of the left IAM demonstrating the facial nerve associated with aplasia of the vestibulocochlear nerve (arrow). **b** T2-weighted high-resolution parasagittal MRI of the IAM demonstrating the facial nerve associated with aplasia of the vestibulocochlear nerve on the right (arrow).

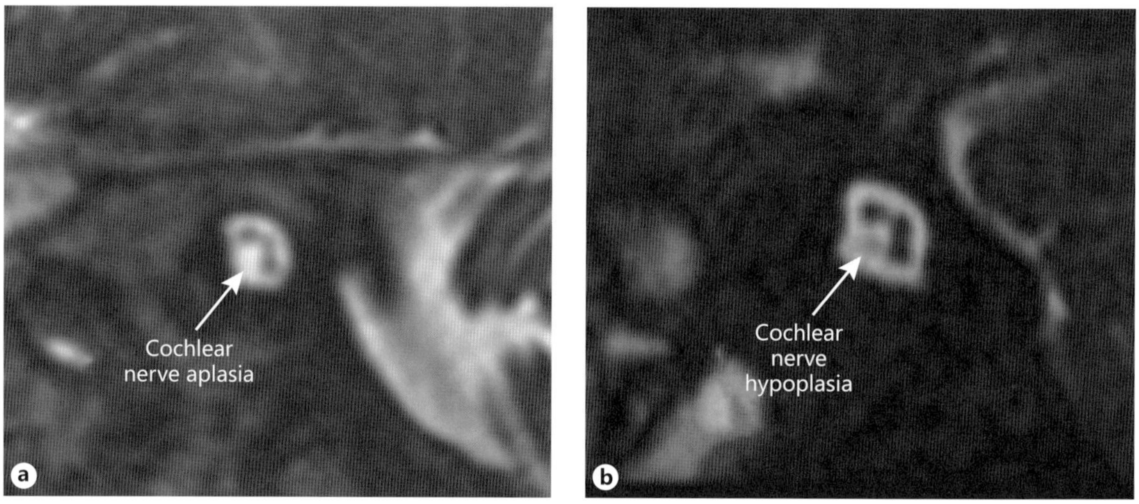

Fig. 3. a, **b** T2-weighted high-resolution parasagittal MRI of the IAM showing cochlear nerve aplasia and hypoplasia.

for example, secondary to patient motion or partial volume averaging. Second, nearby structures such as vascular loops and cerebellar crowding may obscure the nerves. It may not be possible to accurately measure a nerve lying adjacent to the bony wall of the IAC even in a normal temporal bone [14, 15]. Third, CND is often associated with temporal bone malformations. When there is IAC or CNC narrowing, it may be impossible to visualize the CN (Fig. 4). An IEM such as a common cavity may be associated with an unbranching VCN that contains auditory fibres [4]. Finally, it may be possible that the VCN or CN takes an abnormal route in some cases

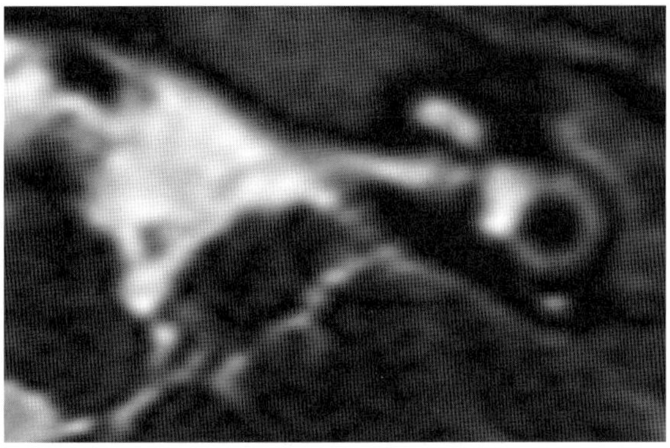

Fig. 4. T2-weighted high-resolution axial MRI demonstrating a very narrow left IAC associated with aplasia of the vestibulocochlear nerve.

and may not be present within the IAC. An absent VCN or CN on MRI should not therefore be a contraindication to CI although benefit is less likely if no nerve is seen [19]. In cases of completely absent IAC, CI benefit has not been reported. Recent improvements in MRI technology including 3 Tesla machines and advanced protocols, are likely to improve the ability to identify the nerve, although it is as yet unclear as to what degree of improvement will be achieved [11, 12].

Audiology

Thai-Van et al. [24] described the case of a child with apparent VCN aplasia who had audiometric thresholds up to 50 dB HL with limited vocalizations. This highlighted the limitations of radiological assessment in cases of CND and that careful audiological assessment should also be performed to fully exclude the presence of auditory neural tissue. A full audiological test battery including both subjective and objective tests should be applied to confirm profound hearing loss [8]. Any repeatable response confirms that auditory nerve fibres must be present, although not necessarily in enough numbers to allow rehabilitation with CI. Responses observed with only low-frequency stimulation at maximum audiometric output should be interpreted with caution as these are usually vibrotactile and may even be present with cochlear aplasia and complete labyrinthine aplasia. In subjective tests, the candidate should be evaluated with insert ear phones. If this is not possible, free field evaluation should be undertaken. According to the age of the child, behavioral observation audiometry, visual reinforced audiometry or play audiometry can be used. Objective evaluation is carried out with tympanometry and acoustic reflex tests to show the middle ear status. These tests should be followed by otoacoustic emissions, and auditory brainstem response (ABR) measurements.

Subjective tests are particularly important even when no response is obtained by other tests and may be the only method that gives information about the hearing status of the patient. Demonstrable behavioral responses with pure tone or speech stimulation despite apparent CN aplasia on MRI signify that the child may benefit from CI. Subjective tests are also helpful for ABI candidacy as an inability to condition to vibrotactile stimulation suggests that, following ABI, programming will be more difficult. Children with severe cognitive impairment are poor ABI candidates because of the difficulties in programming.

Electrical ABR

Casselman et al. [4] noted that the severity of hypoplasia does not necessarily correlate with outcome and recommended that CI assessment for children with CND should include electric promontory stimulation to confirm the functional absence of auditory nerve fibers. Since then, promontory stimulation has been superseded by extracochlear electrical ABR (EABR) measurement and by EABR measurement via intracochlear stimulation through a cochlear implant post-implantation. Several authors have demonstrated that there is good correlation between the quality of the EABR and auditory benefit from implantation in children with CND as determined by speech perception scores [19, 23, 28, 29]. Some false negatives do occur, however, notably due to electrical interference and muscle artefact.

Extracochlear EABR can be used during preoperative assessment, whereby the stimulating electrode is passed transtympanically and placed on the promontory or close to the round window, the latter having reduced impedance. This has been reported to have a high correlation with both intracochlear EABR through the implant and CI benefit. There is probably an element of operator dependence, as demonstrated by variable results and higher false negatives in some centers [19, 30, 31].

An alternative to extracochlear EABR is intracochlear EABR testing using an intracochlear test electrode prior to implantation. Recently, an intracochlear array with 3 electrodes over a length of 18 mm has become available. Although results are as yet unpublished, implant teams from Hacettepe, Manchester and Cambridge have had successful experience with this device and it seems likely to provide similar results to EABR through an implant. It should be noted that, as with other methods of EABR, false negatives may still occur and so decisions regarding CI candidacy should still consider imaging and audiological results as well.

Other Considerations Prior to CI

The age of the child, particularly in relation to consideration of auditory plasticity, is important for candidacy. This is equally important for ABI candidacy in which results are better for children implanted under the age of 3 years [5].

Evaluation Following CI

Once a child has received a cochlear implant, they are closely monitored for 6–9 months to look for signs of progress with auditory perception, using both EABR and behavioral measures. Evoked compound action potentials (ECAP) can also be used, but this test is less reliable in children with CND [17, 19]. Language evaluation by an experienced speech and language therapist is very important. Over the years our teams have observed children with CND who obtained thresholds with CI at 30–40 dB but who do not develop satisfactory speech and language. It is also very important to take the observations of the family into consideration. If there is no development in speech perception and no response on EABR, ABI may be recommended to the family. In this situation, ABI is usually carried out in the contralateral ear, providing bilateral amplification.

CI in CND

With improvements in our understanding of the radiological anatomy and the relationship between outcome from implantation and electrophysiological test results there have been an increasing number of studies reporting outcomes of CI in CND. Broadly speaking, some patients do gain benefit from cochlear implantation but outcomes are generally significantly poorer when compared to patients with normal nerves. Potential predictors of outcome are the presence of some audition preoperatively, the quality of the EABR or ECAP and the presence or absence and size of any VCN or CN present.

Bradley et al. [32] reported their long-term experience in 6 children with hypoplastic CN. These children were implanted preoperatively, and the authors observed clear responses to sound with hearing aids. The IAC was narrow in 4 while 2 had normal width on imaging. On initial programming, all children demonstrated auditory thresholds within the normal range. After 2–6 years of cochlear implant use, however, they demonstrated unsatisfactory outcome: 5 were at level 2 on the Categories of Auditory Perception (CAP) scale [33] and one was at level 4. They concluded that even if they obtained thresholds similar to other CI users, the benefit of CI in children with hypoplastic CN is very limited.

Warren et al. [34] reported CI results in 3 cases with narrow IAC. Patients had 2 visible nerves on MRI; one entering the vestibule in each case while the other was assumed to be the functioning FN. Preoperatively, 2 of the families had reported responses to auditory stimuli with amplification over time. Promontory stimulation testing with electrical stimulation provided positive response in all 3 cases. Although only early postoperative results were available (4, 5 and 9 months respectively), they all showed responses to auditory stimuli. The authors provided 2 possible explanations for sound transmission without any cochlear branch on MRI. The first was that the extremely narrow distal IAC made identification of a thin CN impossible. The second possible explanation was that the nerve turned towards the cochlea after entering the vestibule. Our groups have observed similar cases, where there is a response with implant, sometimes obtaining similar thresholds to implant users with normal anatomy, but progress may hit a ceiling effect, and language development usually does not reach the level achieved in implant recipients with a normal CN.

Valero et al. [35] investigated EABR responses with CI in patients with CND. They observed atypical amplitude and latencies in these patients and suggested that these were likely to be non-auditory in origin. They cautioned that they should not be accepted as typical EABR peaks. Long-term cochlear implant stimulation of the hypoplastic nerve did not promote normal auditory brainstem maturity and did not discourage uncharacteristic development in the brainstem. There was no relationship between the severity of the hypoplastic CN, the diameter of the CNC and IAC and the type of abnormal evoked response. Auditory outcome could not be predicted from the observed evoked responses (in contrast to other authors). They also found that, in spite of initial limited improvement in speech perception, children with CND did not obtain comparable behavioral results with their implants compared to children with normal CN. After long-term use, this difference was still present. These data, along with abnormal electrophysiological findings, support the finding that children with hypoplastic CN do not reach the hearing levels obtained by children with uncompromised CN after CI use.

Buchman et al. [17] reported CI results in patients with inner ear malformations. Their observations were similar to other centers, with poor speech perception in children with CND following CI. They concluded that this is most probably due to insufficient peripheral nerve populations, preventing the development of synchronized auditory stimulation. In these cases, they suggested an initial trial of CI before ABI. They were able to find an association between ECAP testing results and the development of speech perception abilities. They also emphasized the importance of preoperative electrophysiological testing prior to placement of a cochlear implant.

Kutz et al. [18] reported the results of 7 children who underwent CI in an ear without any CN on MRI. One child developed early closed-set speech recognition. The other 6 children developed only speech detection or pattern perception. Two children with hypoplastic nerves were also implanted. One developed consistent closed-set word recognition and the other developed early closed-set word recognition.

Young et al. [20] reported on 10 children with CND receiving a CI. They only implanted children with some measurable auditory responses preoperatively. They found that 1 child developed closed-set recognition and 3 children gained open-set recognition. Although all children had been profoundly deaf, those with slightly better preoperative auditory thresholds, suggesting a greater population of CN fibres, performed better with the cochlear implant.

Yamazaki et al. [16] reported the CI results of 19 children with CND specifically evaluating the importance of VCN size and intracochlear EABR via the implant as predictors of outcome. They found that both factors independently correlated strongly with the postoperative 1 or 2 year CAP score, and if the VCN was hypoplastic and EABR was poor this was an even better predictor of poor outcome. Children with a VCN greater or equal in size to the adjacent FN or with a positive wave V on at least 2 electrodes always gained some benefit with 5 children achieving a CAP 5 or 6. They suggested that these factors could be used to decide early after implantation whether an ABI should be considered.

Recently, Birman et al. [19] reported better outcomes of auditory performance with CI in patients with CND. In the largest study published to date, they implanted 50 children, although 11 of them had unilateral CND only and this latter group was not fully separated out in the results. They classified their results according to the number of nerves seen within the IAC, which correlated with outcome. They also used transtympanic round window EABR preoperatively and found that 98% correlated with the intracochlear EABR via CI, which in turn was present in 96% of implanted ears. ECAP was only found in 40% of implanted ears. Their study found that even when children were diagnosed with CN aplasia on MRI (3 nerves or less seen in the IAC), 50% gained some speech understanding (CAP score 5–7), although only 34% used verbal language as their main mode of communication. In contrast, 90% of those with CN hypoplasia gained CAP 5–7 and 78% used verbal language as their main mode of communication. CN aplasia/hypoplasia was commonly associated with developmental delay and syndromes, particularly CHARGE syndrome. Their findings are encouraging but must be interpreted cautiously given that this level of benefit has not been found by other authors.

ABI in CND

ABI is indicated for children with CND when the assessment process has not demonstrated any evidence that CI might provide benefit or there has been inadequate benefit following CI. ABI is a neurosurgical procedure and carries a risk of serious complications such as cerebrospinal fluid leak, meningitis, intracranial bleeding, stroke, cranial nerve damage and even death. In the hands of experienced teams these risks are low, probably akin to other elective posterior fossa procedures [36]. While a cochlear implant is relatively easy to replace following device failure, replacement of the auditory brainstem implant can be more complicated, with fibrosis of the electrode to the brainstem [37]. Reports of auditory brainstem implant replacements are few, and it remains to be seen how great a problem this will be for the future. Nevertheless, the risks and benefits must be very carefully weighed prior to proceeding.

Colletti et al. [5] were the first to perform this procedure for this indication, and they reported their results with ABI in 59 children, including follow-up of up to 12 years. The study included other indications such as post-meningitis ossification and severe IEMs but the majority had CND. The outcomes were variable, although all children gained some audition. There was a highly significant predictive effect of associated cognitive disorders on auditory outcome with only 9 in 30 achieving environmental sound recognition (CAP 3) and 1 in 30 achieving basic speech recognition (CAP 4). Age (>3 years at implantation) also had a significant effect but children with cognitive disorders were older than those with normal cognition. Overall 90% (26/29) of children with normal cognition were able to recognize environmental sounds, 62% (18/29) gained speech understanding of common phrases without lip reading (CAP 5) and 21% (6/29) could use the telephone with a familiar speaker (CAP 7).

Sennaroglu et al. [6] recently reported the results from Hacettepe regarding ABI in 60 children with complex IEMs and/or CND, with 1 year postoperative results available for 35 children. They demonstrated that all children gained some audition, with the majority of children obtaining CAP scores around category 5. They found a significant correlation with auditory brainstem implant thresholds: better thresholds (25–40 dB) allowed some children to obtain CAP scores of 6, 7 and 8. Unfortunately, speech intelligibility was generally poor with SIR scores of around 2 out of 5, although children with better thresholds obtained scores up to 4. They also found that children with cognitive disorders did significantly worse. Patients with common cavity obtained better scores than other types of IEM in all categories, probably due to the presence of CN fibers. It is possible that bimodal stimulation with CI and ABI may provide better outcomes.

Four other studies have reported their results of prelingually deaf children implanted with an ABI, with a total of 28 children between them [38–41]. These studies have found less successful outcomes: 6 children had no auditory perception and no child achieved a CAP 5 or above. This raises the possibility that there may be important technical aspects to this procedure that are gained with experience.

Sequential CI and ABI in Hypoplastic CN

In Hacettepe University, 83 children underwent ABI surgery between 2006 and 2016: 69 cases have only ABI for hearing restoration and 14 patients use CI and ABI together (unpublished results). These are patients with hypoplastic CN, hypoplastic or incomplete partition type I cochleas and common cavities. When insufficient progress was made following CI over 1 year, a decision for contralateral ABI was made. Some of these children have thresholds of around 40 dB with CI, but because of the hypoplastic CN they show limited progress in language development. An initial analysis of the first 6 patients with sequential CI then ABI was presented in 2015. The mean duration between CI and ABI was 1.5–2 years as the children initially appeared to have acceptable CI thresholds and made progress. When it later became clear a plateau had been reached, ABI was considered. Although they had similar CAP scores in CI only and ABI only situation, auditory performance showed a dramatic increase when CI and ABI were used together. The mean CAP score before ABI was 1, whereas after ABI surgery it was 4.8. A similar improvement was observed in SIR scores as well: before and after ABI mean SIR scores were 1.2 and 3.3, respectively.

Simultaneous CI and ABI

Following the observation that it may take 1–2 years to determine that CI does not provide adequate benefit, the team at Hacettepe started to consider the option of simultaneous CI and ABI. This was done in situations where the outcome with CI is very limited: the CI side has a CN which is barely visible on 3T MRI and there is a very limited response with insert ear phones while the other side has a definite ABI indication. Simultaneous CI and ABI surgeries have 2 advantages. In children who are relatively late for surgery, between 2–3 years, waiting for the result of CI surgery may result in late ABI surgery. Additional disabilities may make it more difficult to decide whether the child is making progress with CI, which also results in delayed ABI surgery. When the child approaches 3–4 years of age, the benefit from ABI decreases. To avoid this, CI and ABI can be done in the same setting. If the child benefits from CI, then they will have bilateral stimulation at the start. In cases where CI is not beneficial, the child will not lose valuable time waiting for ABI. This approach has been used in 2 patients so far in Hacettepe (unpublished results).

Clinical Pathway

Figure 5 shows the clinical pathway undertaken by patients with CND in Manchester. This is based on recommendations made at the second consensus meeting on hypoplastic and aplastic VCN and highlights the importance of

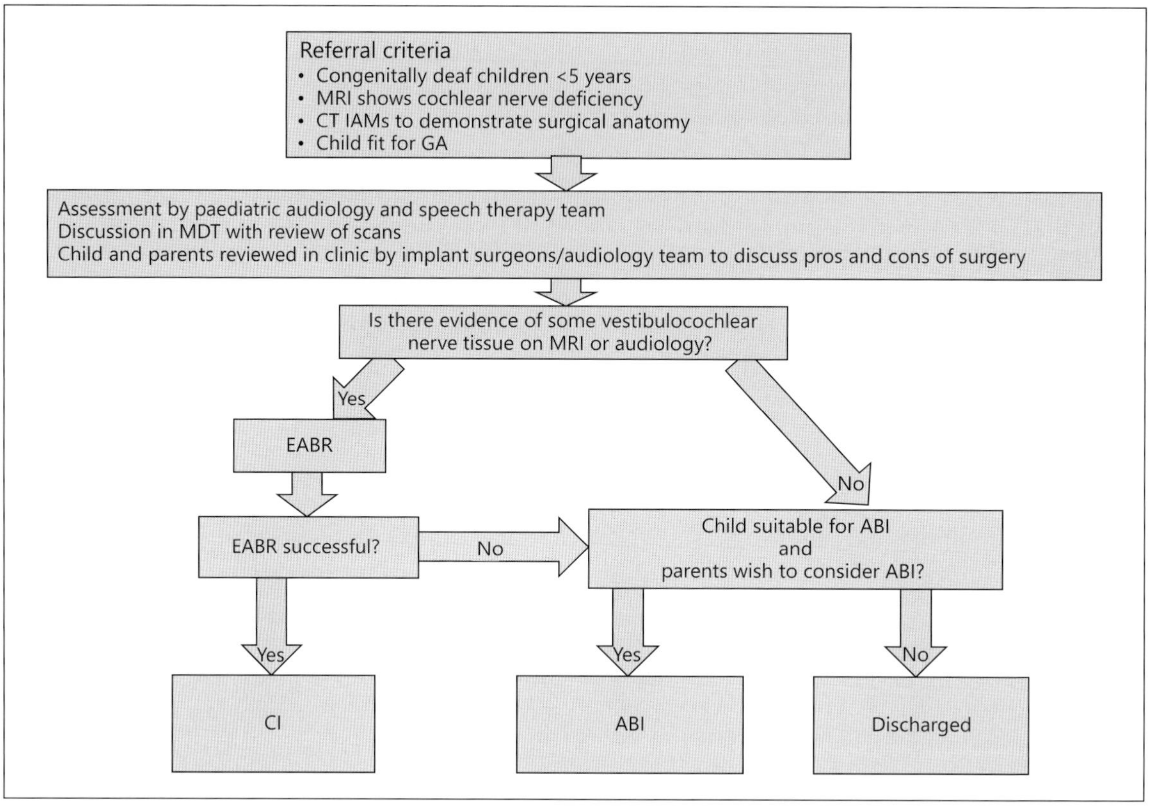

Fig. 5. Flow chart demonstrating the patient pathway for investigation and management of VCN/CN hypoplasia/aplasia.

a multidisciplinary approach. The decision-making process is complex. The most challenging areas within this pathway are:

1. Optimizing the radiological process and interpretation of the results.

2. Determining whether or not an EABR is present and, if so, of what quality?

3. Whether or not the patients wish their child to be considered for implantation with uncertain outcome. This is particularly true of those being considered for ABI.

4. The presence of significant learning difficulties in association with the VCN/CN abnormalities. Again, this is particularly important for those being considered for ABI as programming the device in the presence of significant learning difficulties is extremely challenging.

Conclusion

Even with today's technology, it is very difficult to predict the best treatment modality in patients with CND. Radiological and audiological evaluation methods are not yet precise enough to let the clinician decide between CI and ABI. CI is usually not promising, often resulting in poor outcomes with CAP scores <5. ABI may provide better outcomes but at the expense of a more serious operation with greater risks and the possibility that device replacement may be complicated. When possible these candidates should be given the option of CI first and then ABI. A minority of patients presenting late (around 2–3 years of age) may be candidates for simultaneous CI and ABI.

References

1 Kaplan AB, Kozin ED, Puram SV, Owoc MS, Shah PV, Hight AE, Sethi RKV, Remenschneider AK, Lee DJ: Auditory brainstem implant candidacy in the United States in children 0-17 years old. Int J Pediatr Otorhinolaryngol 2015;79: 310–315.

2 Jackler RK, Luxford WM, House WF: Congenital malformations of the inner ear: a classification based on embryogenesis. Laryngoscope 1987;97(3 pt 2 suppl 40):2–14.

3 Shelton C, Luxford WM, Tonokawa LL, Lo WW, House WF: The narrow internal auditory canal in children: a contraindication to cochlear implants. Otolaryngol Head Neck Surg 1989;100: 227–231.

4 Casselman JW, Offeciers FE, Govaerts PJ, Kuhweide R, Geldof H, Somers T, D'Hont G: Aplasia and hypoplasia of the vestibulocochlear nerve: diagnosis with MR imaging. Radiology 1997;202:773–781.

5 Colletti L, Shannon RV, Colletti V: The development of auditory perception in children after auditory brainstem implantation. Audiol Neurootol 2014;19: 386–394.

6 Sennaroğlu L, Sennaroğlu G, Yücel E, Bilginer B, Atay G, Bajin MD, Mocan BÖ, Yaral M, Aslan F, Çnar BÇ, Özkan B, Batuk MÖ, Kirazl ÇE, Karakaya J, Ataş A, Saraç S, Ziyal İ: Long-term results of ABI in children with severe inner ear malformations. Otol Neurotol 2016;37:865–872.

7 Sennaroglu L, Colletti V, Manrique M, Laszig R, Offeciers E, Saeed S, Ramsden R, Sarac S, Freeman S, Andersen HR, Zarowski A, Ziyal I, Sollmann WP, Kaminsky J, Bejarano B, Atas A, Sennaroglu G, Yucel E, Sevinc S, Colletti L, Huarte A, Henderson L, Wesarg T, Konradsson K: Auditory brainstem implantation in children and non-neurofibromatosis type 2 patients: a consensus statement. Otol Neurotol 2011;32:187–191.

8 Sennaroğlu L, Colletti V, Lenarz T, Manrique M, Laszig R, Rask-Andersen H, Göksu N, Offeciers E, Saeed S, Behr R, Bayazıt Y, Casselman J, Freeman S, Kileny P, Lee DJ, Shannon RV, Kameswaran M, Hagr A, Zarowski A, Schwartz MS, Bilginer B, Kishore A, Sennaroğlu G, Yücel E, Saraç S, Ataş A, Colletti L, O'Driscoll M, Moon IS, Gärtner L, Huarte A, Nyberg G, Mocan BÖ, Atay G, Bajin MD, Çınar BÇ, Batuk MÖ, Yaralı M, Aydınlı FE, Aslan F, Kirazlı MC, Özkan HB, Hans JM, Kosaner J, Polak M: Consensus statement: long-term results of ABI in children with complex inner ear malformations and decision making between CI and ABI. Cochlear Implants Int 2016;17:163–171.

9 Adunka OF, Roush PA, Teagle HF, Brown CJ, Zdanski CJ, Jewells V, Buchman CA: Internal auditory canal morphology in children with cochlear nerve deficiency. Otol Neurotol 2006;27:793–801.

10 Adunka OF, Jewells V, Buchman CA: Value of computed tomography in the evaluation of children with cochlear nerve deficiency. Otol Neurotol 2007;28: 597–604.

11 Noij KS, Remenschneider AK, Kozin ED, Puram S, Herrmann B, Cohen M, Cunnane MB, Lee DJ: Direct parasagittal magnetic resonance imaging of the internal auditory canal to determine cochlear or auditory brainstem implant candidacy in children. Laryngoscope 2015;125:2382–2385.

12 Giesemann AM, Raab P, Lyutenski S, Dettmer S, Bültmann E, Frömke C, Lenarz T, Lanfermann H, Goetz F: Improved imaging of cochlear nerve hypoplasia using a 3-Tesla variable flip-angle turbo spin-echo sequence and a 7-cm surface coil. Laryngoscope 2014;124: 751–754.

13 Kim HS, Kim DI, Chung IH, Lee WS, Kim KY: Topographical relationship of the facial and vestibulocochlear nerves in the subarachnoid space and internal auditory canal. AJNR Am J Neuroradiol 1998;19:1155–1161.

14 Nakamichi R, Yamazaki M, Ikeda M, Isoda H, Kawai H, Sone M, Nakashima T, Naganawa S: Establishing normal diameter range of the cochlear and facial nerves with 3D-CISS at 3T. Magn Reson Med Sci 2013;12:241–247.

15 Jaryszak EM, Patel NA, Camp M, Mancuso AA, Antonelli PJ: Cochlear nerve diameter in normal hearing ears using high-resolution magnetic resonance imaging. Laryngoscope 2009;119:2042–2045.

16 Yamazaki H, Leigh J, Briggs R, Naito Y: Usefulness of MRI and EABR testing for predicting CI outcomes immediately after cochlear implantation in cases with cochlear nerve deficiency. Otol Neurotol 2015;36:977–984.

17 Buchman CA, Teagle HF, Roush PA, Park LR, Hatch D, Woodard J, Zdanski C, Adunka OF: Cochlear implantation in children with labyrinthine anomalies and cochlear nerve deficiency: implications for auditory brainstem implantation. Laryngoscope 2011;121:1979–1988.

18 Kutz JW Jr, Lee KH, Isaacson B, Booth TN, Sweeney MH, Roland PS: Cochlear implantation in children with cochlear nerve absence or deficiency. Otol Neurotol 2011;32:956–961.

19 Birman CS, Powell HR, Gibson WP, Elliott EJ: Cochlear implant outcomes in cochlea nerve aplasia and hypoplasia. Otol Neurotol 2016;37:438–445.

20 Young NM, Kim FM, Ryan ME, Tournis E, Yaras S: Pediatric cochlear implantation of children with eighth nerve deficiency. Int J Pediatr Otorhinolaryngol 2012;76:1442–1448.

21 Levi J, Ames J, Bacik K, Drake C, Morlet T, O'Reilly RC: Clinical characteristics of children with cochlear nerve dysplasias. Laryngoscope 2013;123:752–756.

22 Clemmens CS, Guidi J, Caroff A, Cohn SJ, Brant JA, Laury AM, Bilaniuk LT, Germiller JA: Unilateral cochlear nerve deficiency in children. Otolaryngol Head Neck Surg 2013;149:318–325.

23 Song MH, Kim SC, Kim J, Chang JW, Lee WS, Choi JY: The cochleovestibular nerve identified during auditory brainstem implantation in patients with narrow internal auditory canals: can preoperative evaluation predict cochleovestibular nerve deficiency? Laryngoscope 2011;121:1773–1779.

24 Thai-Van H, Fraysse B, Berry I, Berges C, Deguine O, Honegger A, Sevely A, Ibarrola D: Functional magnetic resonance imaging may avoid misdiagnosis of cochleovestibular nerve aplasia in congenital deafness. Am J Otol 2000;21: 663–670.
25 Casselman JW, Offeciers EF, De Foer B, Govaerts P, Kuhweide R, Somers T: CT and MR imaging of congential abnormalities of the inner ear and internal auditory canal. Eur J Radiol 2001;40: 94–104.
26 Giesemann AM, Raab P, Lyutenski S, Dettmer S, Bültmann E, Frömke C, Lenarz T, Lanfermann H, Goetz F: Improved imaging of cochlear nerve hypoplasia using a 3-Tesla variable flip-angle turbo spin-echo sequence and a 7-cm surface coil. Laryngoscope 2014;124: 751–754.
27 Freeman SR, Stivaros SM, Ramsden RT, O'Driscoll MP, Nichani JR, Bruce IA, Green KM, Henderson LA, Rutherford SA, King AT, Lloyd SK: The management of cochlear nerve deficiency. Cochlear Implants Int 2013;14(suppl 4): S27–S31.
28 Song MH, Bae MR, Kim HN, Lee WS, Yang WS, Choi JY: Value of intracochlear electrically evoked auditory brainstem response after cochlear implantation in patients with narrow internal auditory canal. Laryngoscope 2010;120: 1625–1631.
29 Walton J, Gibson WP, Sanli H, Prelog K: Predicting cochlear implant outcomes in children with auditory neuropathy. Otol Neurotol 2008;29:302–309.
30 Kim AH, Kileny PR, Arts HA, El-Kashlan HK, Telian SA, Zwolan TA: Role of electrically evoked auditory brainstem response in cochlear implantation of children with inner ear malformations. Otol Neurotol 2008;29:626–634.
31 Mason SM, O'Donoghue GM, Gibbin KP, Garnham CW, Jowett CA: Perioperative electrical auditory brain stem response in candidates for pediatric cochlear implantation. Am J Otol 1997;18: 466–471.
32 Bradley J, Beale T, Graham J, Bell M: Variable long-term outcomes from cochlear implantation in children with hypoplastic auditory nerves. Cochlear Implants Int 2008;9:34–60.
33 Archbold S, Lutman ME, Marshall DH: Categories of auditory performance. Ann Otol Rhinol Laryngol Suppl 1995; 166:312–314.
34 Warren FM 3rd, Wiggins RH 3rd, Pitt C, Harnsberger HR, Shelton C: Apparent cochlear nerve aplasia: to implant or not to implant? Otol Neurotol 2010;31: 1088–1094.
35 Valero J, Blaser S, Papsin BC, James AL, Gordon KA: Electrophysiologic and behavioral outcomes of cochlear implantation in children with auditory nerve hypoplasia. Ear Hear 2012;33:3–18.
36 Colletti V, Shannon RV, Carner M, Veronese S, Colletti L: Complications in auditory brainstem implant surgery in adults and children. Otol Neurotol 2010; 31:558–564.
37 Ramsden RT, Freeman SR, Lloyd SK, King AT, Shi X, Ward CL, Huson SM, Mawman DJ, O'Driscoll MP, Evans DG, Rutherford SA; Manchester Neurofibromatosis Type 2 Service: Auditory brainstem implantation in neurofibromatosis type 2: experience from the manchester programme. Otol Neurotol 2016;37: 1267–1274.
38 Siegbahn M, Lundin K, Olsson GB, Stillesjö F, Kinnefors A, Rask-Andersen H, Nyberg G: Auditory brainstem implants (ABIs) – 20 years of clinical experience in Uppsala, Sweden. Acta Otolaryngol 2014;134:1052–1061.
39 Bayazit YA, Kosaner J, Cinar BC, Atac A, Tutar H, Gunduz B, Altinyay S, Gokdogan C, Ant A, Ozdek A, Goksu N: Methods and preliminary outcomes of pediatric auditory brainstem implantation. Ann Otol Rhinol Laryngol 2014;123: 529–536.
40 Bento RF, Monteiro TA, Tsuji RK, Gomez MQ, Hausen Pinna M, Goffi-Gomez MV, Brito R: Retrolabyrinthine approach for surgical placement of auditory brainstem implants in children. Acta Otolaryngol 2012;132:462–466.
41 Choi JY, Song MH, Jeon JH, Lee WS, Chang JW: Early surgical results of auditory brainstem implantation in nontumor patients. Laryngoscope 2011;121: 2610–2618.

Mr. Simon R. Freeman
Department of Otolaryngology, Peter Mount Building, Manchester Royal Infirmary
Oxford Road
Manchester, M13 9WL (UK)
E-Mail simon.freeman@cmft.nhs.uk

Lloyd SKW, Donnelly NP (eds): Advances in Hearing Rehabilitation.
Adv Otorhinolaryngol. Basel, Karger, 2018, vol 81, pp 93–104 (DOI: 10.1159/000485526)

Hearing Rehabilitation in Neurofibromatosis Type 2

Hannah J.D. North[a] · Simon K.W. Lloyd[b]

[a]Westmead Hospital, Sydney, NSW, Australia; [b]University Department of Otolaryngology Head and Neck Surgery, Peter Mount House, Manchester Royal Infirmary, Manchester, UK

Abstract

Bilateral vestibular schwannomas are almost pathognomonic of neurofibromatosis type 2 (NF2). As a result of these tumors, hearing loss is the presenting symptom in 60% of adults and 30% of children with NF2. It is often bilateral. The best means of preserving hearing in patients with NF2 is conservative management. Even so at least 28% of patients have progression of hearing loss following diagnosis. The likelihood of progression of hearing loss is, at least in part, determined by the type of mutation. Treatment of vestibular schwannomas often has a detrimental effect on hearing. Only 41% of patients having stereotactic radiosurgery maintain their hearing at 5 years. Treatment with bevacizumab maintains medium-term hearing in 38% and improves it in 48%. Surgery to remove vestibular schwannomas invariably leads to complete loss of ipsilateral hearing, although in a very limited number of patients hearing preservation surgery may be possible. For those that lose their hearing but have an intact cochlear nerve, for example, conservative management, radiotherapy treatment or cochlear nerve preserving surgery, cochlear implantation has been shown to be an effective option although outcomes are not as good as traditional implant candidates (mean sentence testing scores in quiet: stable untreated tumors 69%; radiotherapy treated tumors 49%; cochlear nerve preserving surgery ~40%). For those that do not have a functional cochlear nerve, auditory brainstem implantation (ABI) is an option. The non-user rate in this group is 13%. The mean sentence score in users with ABI alone is 12%. ABI therefore acts, in most cases, as an aid to lip reading and rarely provides open set speech discrimination.

Introduction

Hearing loss is one of the main factors influencing the quality of life in patients with neurofibromatosis type 2 (NF2) [1–3]. It is almost inevitable either as a result of the presence of bilateral vestibular schwannoma or its treatment. Its effects are more devastating in NF2 compared to those with sporadic unilateral vestibular schwannomas because of the hearing loss is often bilateral rather than unilateral.

Decision making around hearing preservation or rehabilitation in patients with NF2 is complex. It must be balanced with the need for tumor control in the presence of an often aggressive disease

Table 1. AAO-HNS categories of hearing loss

	AAO-HNS hearing classification			
	serviceable hearing		non-serviceable	
	A	B	C	D
PTA, dB	<30	30–50	>50	Any
SDS, %	>70	50–70	>50	<50

AAO-HNS, American Academy of Otorhinolaryngologists Head and Neck Surgeons; PTA, pure tone audiometry; SDS, speech discrimination testing.

Table 2. UK NF2 consensus group grading system for the assessment of hearing loss in NF2

Grade	Test	Deficit
1	>70% SDS in better hearing ear	Normal or near normal hearing with or without acoustic hearing aids
2	50–69% SDS in better hearing ear	Good benefit from acoustic hearing aids
3	<50% SDS in better hearing ear; ≥50% BKB	Adequate benefit from acoustic hearing aids, best-aided condition
4	<50%SDS in better hearing ear; <50% BKB	Poor benefit from acoustic hearing aids, consider auditory implant
5	Auditory implant	
6	Dead ear	

Speech discrimination score (SDS) is the percentage of phonemes within 10 monosyllabic words correctly identified at an optimal sound intensity. Bamford-Kowal-Bench (BKB) standard sentence lists comprise 21 lists, each having 16 sentences and 50 keywords (3 or 4 per sentence) presented at an optimal sound intensity.

and with the potential risk of a given intervention. This is made more complicated by the fact that both ears must be taken into consideration.

In the past 25 years, the hearing rehabilitation options available to clinicians have expanded considerably, particularly with the introduction of less invasive treatments such as chemotherapy and the availability of electrical stimulation of the cochlear nerve with cochlear implantation and of the cochlear nucleus with auditory brainstem implantation (ABI).

The following chapter summarizes the current evidence base behind the management options available to patients with NF2.

The Natural History of Hearing in NF2

Outcome Measurements of Hearing Loss

Most clinicians use the American Academy of Otorhinolaryngologists Head and Neck Surgeons (AAO-HNS) hearing classification system to categorize the severity of hearing loss (Table 1). This in turn can determine the hearing rehabilitation recommendations. A consensus document on the evaluation of hearing loss in NF2 has been published by the UK NF2 group (Table 2) [4]. In the UK, it is recommended that patients with NF2 should have an annual pure tone audiometry and speech discrimination test-

Table 3. Minimum documentation recommended in patients with NF2

For all cases
Mean tumor size at treatment (this should be recorded according to CPA component and, where possible as a volume in cm^3)
Annual tumor growth
Mean tumor size at last follow-up, if relevant
Completeness of tumor removal, if relevant
Radiological recurrence rate, if relevant
Duration of follow-up (this should ideally be at least 5 years)
For hearing preservation interventions
Pure tone and speech discrimination data prior to commencement of treatment and at last follow-up according to AAO-HNS recommendations. As well as SDS at 40 dB, the maximum SDS and the sound intensity at which it is achieved should also be recorded
Proportion maintaining serviceable hearing (defined as AAO-HNS class A or B)
Tumor control (this should be defined as no change in size within 2 mm of pre-treatment scan on imaging not as no intervention)
For radiotherapy, technique used and marginal/maximum radiation dose
For auditory implantation
Speech discrimination scores with and without lip reading in quiet and in noise with sentences delivered at 70 dB
For patients with poor outcomes, word scores and environmental sound awareness assessment
Implant user
Use of telephone

ing (SDS) with Arthur Bothroyd words. If required, annual hearing aid assessments are also undertaken to ensure hearing is optimized. Once SDS is <50%, annual Bamford-Kowal-Bench (BKB) sentence testing is undertaken. This should be performed in best aided conditions and with optimum sound intensity, as determined by the SDS. BKB sentence scores of <50% indicate that the patient is struggling with conventional hearing aids and should then be assessed for auditory implantation. Plotkin et al. [5] have put forward a consensus statement on reporting hearing and tumor treatment outcomes in patients with NF2 (Table 3).

It is important to note that, because of the bilateral nature of NF2 vestibular schwannomas, it is likely that class C or even good class D hearing will be helpful if the contralateral ear is profoundly deaf, and this should be taken into consideration when making management decisions that could potentially affect residual hearing.

Hearing at Presentation

Hearing loss in patients with NF2 is most commonly attributed to vestibular schwannomas, although it may result from cochlear schwannomas, cerebellopontine angle (CPA) meningiomas or middle ear dysfunction from middle fossa meningiomas. The degree of hearing loss at presentation varies in patients with vestibular schwannomas. Historically, hearing loss has been common at initial presentation, occurring in 60% of adults and 30% of children [6]. Surprisingly, more recent prospective studies show a large proportion of patients with no or minimal hearing loss at presentation. For example, Plotkin et al. [7] found that 71% of patients with NF2 have no hearing loss at presentation (AAO class A). It is probable that this difference relates to a higher proportion of patients being diagnosed early with milder phenotypes and smaller tumors as a result of improvements in imaging and screening protocols. When hearing loss is present at presentation, it is often unilateral. Peyre et al. [8] found that 85% of patients with NF2 had serviceable hearing in at least one ear at presentation.

Deterioration of Hearing
With time, hearing loss often progresses to a bilateral hearing loss, although this may remain asymmetrical [6]. This hearing loss may be gradual, stepwise or sudden, with between 5 and 15% having sudden hearing loss [9, 10]. In Plotkin's patient group [5], 28% of patients experienced hearing decline (defined as an increase in threshold of >6 dB) over a median period of 62 months. Five percent had a hearing decline at 1 year, 13% had a hearing decline at 2 years and 16% had a hearing decline at 3 years. Around 16% of ears experienced hearing improvement. The NF2 Natural History Consortium found that 27% of patients had a deterioration in hearing over a 2 year period [11].

Sudden deterioration in hearing should be assessed as a matter of urgency with consideration of oral or intra-tympanic corticosteroids.

Hearing Deterioration Related to Tumor Growth
Hearing loss may be sensory, neural or a combination of the two. It results from impaired vascular supply to the cochlea or the cochlear nerve, direct invasion of the cochlea or cochlear nerve by tumor or from proteinaceous deposition within the cochlea [10]. Tumor type in the CPA has anecdotally been noted to affect hearing loss with meningiomas causing less hearing loss than similar sized vestibular schwannomas. Reports of hearing deterioration in relation to tumor growth alone are controversial. Some groups have found that there was no correlation between change in hearing threshold and tumor growth [9, 12]. In contrast, Lalwani et al. [13] found that there was a correlation between greater tumor size at presentation and poorer hearing threshold. Hearing loss in one ear does not appear to be correlated with hearing loss in the second ear [12].

Genetic Severity to Predict the Rate of Hearing Loss
Disease severity may have a negative correlation with hearing outcome. Conversely, smaller size, younger age at surgery and family history of NF2 may be associated with better hearing outcomes [14, 15]. Evans et al. [16] have recently described different patterns in genetic severity of disease load in NF2 that can be roughly divided into mild, moderate and severe genetic clusters, and it may be that these genotypes correlate with hearing phenotype.

Treatment of Tumors and Their Effects on Hearing

Most of the literature regarding hearing outcomes with different treatment modalities consists of small- or medium-sized case series and do not take into consideration other factors that could potentially influence hearing results. These include tumor size, tumor behavior, patient age, patient comorbidities, presence of multiple CPA tumors, tumor cysts, cochlear involvement with tumor, patient preference and local expertise. In addition, there are no control groups and much of the literature only reports short- or medium-term hearing outcomes. Similarly, there are no studies comparing hearing outcomes in patients receiving radiotherapy, undergoing conservative management or having hearing preservation surgery. Care, therefore, needs to be taken in interpreting the literature.

Radiotherapy and Its Effect on Hearing
Radiotherapy is a widely accepted means of treating growing sporadic vestibular schwannomas smaller than around 25 mm in diameter. Tumor control rates appear to be between 80 and 100% depending on the series, but control appears lower in NF2. Hearing outcomes following radiotherapy, particularly long term, have generally been poorly reported. It is also unclear how much of the observed hearing loss over time is treatment related or related to natural progression of hearing

loss. There are also few studies directly comparing hearing outcomes between different types of radiotherapy options, including conventional fractionated radiotherapy, hypofractionated radiotherapy and stereotactic radiosurgery (SRS). Several case studies document hearing outcomes in particular radiotherapy regimes [17–29], but only five of these include follow-up out to 5 years.

Stereotactic Radiosurgery
Meta-analysis of studies examining SRS shows that under half (mean 41.1%) of patients maintained serviceable hearing over a mean follow-up period of 58 months [17–25]. The dosage varied between series and often varied over time with patients earlier in the series tending to have received higher doses than more recently treated patients. The dosage was reduced over time because of an awareness of the relatively poor hearing outcomes from higher doses [18, 20, 21]. In some series, a significant proportion of patients had had previous surgery on the tumor being treated [17, 20, 30].

Fractionated Radiotherapy
Fractionated radiotherapy appears to have slightly better hearing preservation outcomes over a similar period (57.3%) [27, 28], but this conclusion should be interpreted with care because of the low number of patients in the fractionated radiotherapy cohort. No reliable conclusions can be drawn with regards to hearing outcomes with hypofractionated radiotherapy because of the very low numbers of patients treated in this way.

Chemotherapy and Its Effects on Hearing
Since 2009, Bevacizumab has become increasingly used to control vestibular schwannoma growth in NF2. It is a monoclonal antibody of vascular endothelial growth factor A that acts through the inhibition of angiogenesis. Initial short- to medium-term results show it to have a positive influence on hearing as well as a significant reduction in the number of patients requiring definitive treatment either surgery or radiotherapy for their growing tumors. The dose used varies between different units and countries but over a mean follow-up period of 21 months, 38.3% of patients had stable hearing on treatment and 48.3% of patients appear to have an improvement in their hearing. The median improvement in word score recognition was 10% but the extent of the response was highly variable and ranged from –44 to 89% [31–37].

Other drugs have also been trialed including Erlotinib (estimated glomerular filtration rate antagonist) [38], Imatinib (tyrosine kinase inhibitor), Evorilimus (an immunosuppressant and a derivative of serolimus) [39], Lapatinib (tyrosine kinase inhibitor) [40] and Pazopanib (tyrosine kinase inhibitor) [35]. These have not entered routine clinical practice because of lack of efficacy or significant side effects.

Surgery and Its Effect on Hearing
Surgery for tumors in the CPA is generally via one of 3 approaches – 2 are potentially hearing preserving approaches with the potential to preserve the cochlear, vestibular and cochlear nerves: the retrosigmoid approach and the middle cranial fossa approach. The third approach is the translabyrinthine approach and does not allow preservation of hearing, but has the potential to preserve the cochlea and cochlear nerve which may allow hearing rehabilitation using a cochlear implant either simultaneously or at a later date. The choice of surgical approach depends on multiple factors including ipsilateral preoperative hearing, tumor type (vestibular schwannoma, meningioma, other schwannoma or other tumor), tumor size, the presence of cerebrospinal fluid in the internal auditory canal, surgeon preference, and most importantly in NF2, the presence of collision tumors.

Retrosigmoid Approach
Only one unit [41, 42] has looked specifically at hearing outcomes using the retrosigmoid approach. They attempted to preserve hearing in all patients (including tumors up to 50 mm) accessed

65 Arístegui M, Denia A: Simultaneous cochlear implantation and translabyrinthine removal of vestibular schwannoma in an only hearing ear: report of 2 cases (neurofibromatosis type 2 and unilateral vestibular schwannoma). Otol Neurotol 2005;26:205–210.
66 Hoffman RA, Kohan D, Cohen NL: Cochlear implants in the management of bilateral acoustic neuromas. Am J Otol 1992;13:525–528.
67 Lassaletta L, Aristegui M, Medina M, Aranguez G, Pérez-Mora RM, Falcioni M, et al: Ipsilateral cochlear implantation in patients with sporadic vestibular schwannoma in the only or best hearing ear and in patients with NF2. Eur Arch Otorhinolaryngol 2016;273:27–35.
68 Goddard JC, Schwartz MS, Friedman RA: Fundal fluid as a predictor of hearing preservation in the middle cranial fossa approach for vestibular schwannoma. Otol Neurotol 2010;31:1128–1134.
69 Celis-Aguilar E, Lassaletta L, Gavilán J: Cochlear implantation in patients with neurofibromatosis type 2 and patients with vestibular schwannoma in the only hearing ear. Int J Otolaryngol 2012;2012: 157497.
70 Colletti L, Shannon R, Colletti V: Auditory brainstem implants for neurofibromatosis type 2. Curr Opin Otolaryngol Head Neck Surg 2012;20:353–357.
71 Maini S, Cohen MA, Hollow R, Briggs R: Update on long-term results with auditory brainstem implants in NF2 patients. Cochlear Implants Int 2009; 10(suppl 1):33–37.
72 Briggs RJ, Fagan P, Atlas M, Kaye AH, Sheehy J, Hollow R, Shaw S, Clark GM: Multichannel auditory brainstem implantation: the Australian experience. J Laryngol Otol Suppl 2000;27:46–49.
73 Lenarz T, Moshrefi M, Matthies C, Frohne C, Lesinski-Schiedat A, Illg A, et al: Auditory Brainstem Implant: part I. Auditory performance and its evolution over time. Otol Neurotol 2001;22:823–833.
74 Kalamarides M, Grayeli AB, Bouccara D, et al: Hearing restoration with auditory brainstem implants after radiosurgery for neurofibromatosis Type 2. J Neurosurg 2001;95:1028–1033.
75 Otto SR, Brackmann DE, Hitselberger WE, Shannon RV, Kuchta J: Multichannel auditory brainstem implant: update on performance in 61 patients. J Neurosurg 2002;96:1063–1071.
76 Nevison B, Laszig R, Sollmann WP, Lenarz T, Sterkers O, Ramsden R, et al: Results from a European clinical investigation of the nucleus multichannel auditory brainstem implant. Ear Hear 2002; 23:170–183.
77 Behr R, Colletti V, Matthies C, Morita A, Nakatomi H, Dominique L, et al: New outcomes with auditory brainstem implants in NF2 patients. Otol Neurotol 2014;35:1844–1851.
78 Kanowitz SJ, Shapiro WH, Golfinos JG, Cohen NL, Roland JT Jr: Auditory brainstem implantation in patients with neurofibromatosis type 2. Laryngoscope 2004;114:2135–2146.
79 Grayeli AB, Kalamarides M, Bouccara D, Ambert-Dahan E, Sterkers O: Auditory brainstem implant in neurofibromatosis type 2 and non-neurofibromatosis type 2 patients. Otol Neurotol 2008;29:1140–1146.
80 Goffi-Gomez MV, Magalhães AT, Brito Neto R, Tsuji RK, Gomes Mde Q, Bento RF: Auditory brainstem implant outcomes and MAP parameters: report of experiences in adults and children. Int J Pediatr Otorhinolaryngol 2012;76:257–264.
81 Sanna M, Di Lella F, Guida M, Merkus P: Auditory brainstem implants in NF2 patients: results and review of the literature. Otol Neurotol 2012;33:154–164.
82 Monteiro TA, Goffi-Gomez MV, Tsuji RK, et al: Neurofibromatosis 2: hearing restoration options. Braz J Otorhinolaryngol 2012;78:128–134.
83 Ramsden RT, Freeman SR, Lloyd SK, King AT, Shi X, Ward CL, Huson SM, Mawman DJ, O'Driscoll MP, Evans DG, Rutherford SA; Manchester Neurofibromatosis Type 2 Service: Auditory brainstem implantation in neurofibromatosis type 2: experience from the Manchester programme. Otol Neurotol 2016;37: 1267–1274.
84 McSorley A, Freeman SR, Ramsden RT, Motion J, King AT, Rutherford SA, et al: Subjective outcomes of auditory brainstem implantation. Otol Neurotol 2015; 36:873–878.
85 Otto SR, Shannon RV, Wilkinson EP, Hitselberger WE, McCreery DB, Moore JK, Brackmann DE: Audiologic outcomes with the penetrating electrode auditory brainstem implant. Otol Neurotol 2008;29:1147–1154.
86 Lenarz T, Lim HH, Reuter G, Patrick JF, Lenarz M: The auditory midbrain implant: a new auditory prosthesis for neural deafness-concept and device description. Otol Neurotol 2006;27:838–843.

Prof. Simon K.W. Lloyd
University Department of Otolaryngology Head and Neck Surgery
Peter Mount House, Manchester Royal Infirmary
Oxford Road
Manchester M13 9WL (UK)
E-Mail sklloyd@me.com

Lloyd SKW, Donnelly NP (eds): Advances in Hearing Rehabilitation.
Adv Otorhinolaryngol. Basel, Karger, 2018, vol 81, pp 105–113 (DOI: 10.1159/000485540)

The Future of Cochlear Implant Design

Alistair Mitchell-Innes[a] · Shakeel R. Saeed[b] · Richard Irving[a]

[a]University Hospital Birmingham, Birmingham, and [b]University College London, London, UK

Abstract

This chapter discusses the multifaceted future of cochlear implant design. Current research is focused on novel strategies relating to the electrode array, aiming to improve the neuronal health and spatial selectivity, and reduce the power consumption. Future design iterations will most likely improve the neuronal health by reducing insertion trauma, minimizing the inflammatory pathway that follows electrode insertion or through the use of neurotrophins or stem cells. Improvements in spatial selectivity and in speech recognition in difficult listening environments can be achieved through changes in the electrode/neural interface. Designing an array that brings the electrodes closer to neural tissue, or changing the method of stimulation with current steering or even optical or piezoelectric stimulation are discussed. Increasing the MRI compatibility is an important consideration, and devices allowing remote programming have a huge impact on worldwide provision. Technology exists to realize the elusive goal of a fully implantable cochlear implant, allowing continuous and invisible hearing. Ultimately, future technologies will be integrated to allow tailoring of implant design to the individual, thereby addressing the broad variability in user performance. At the same time, there is an urgent requirement for a high quality, low cost, mass-produced implant for the developing world.

Introduction

Cochlear implants have evolved from bulky, body-worn single electrode technologies in the 1960s, to the multi-channel ear level or single unit devices that exist today. Multiple iterations of speech processing strategies and electrode arrays now enable many users to achieve speech reception in quiet up to the level of normal listeners. Current devices, however, confer limited ability to appreciate music and often do not perform well in a noisy environment or offer optimal sound localization. Those who use tonal language often also have more limited benefits from implantation. Therefore, there is still significant scope for improving the function. Similarly, whilst implants have become progressively smaller and more discrete, there is still a need to wear an external processor. The aim of future technological developments is therefore to provide hearing outcomes comparable to natural hearing from a fully implantable device that would allow both "continuous" and "hidden" hearing. Ultimately, it is likely that implant design will allow customization to the individual, thereby addressing the broad variability in user performance. There is also an urgent need for a high quality, low cost, mass-produced implant for the developing world as current devices are expensive. This together with a lack of public awareness, absence of new born screening programs and poor accessibility to diagnostic centers means that the availability of cochlear implants in the developing world is very limited [1, 2]. Combining this technology with remote programming of the speech processing software would allow more effective hearing rehabilitation. This chapter provides a summary of current and future research aimed at achieving the above goals.

Recent Changes in Speech Processing

The advent of multi-channel devices in the early 1980s allowed subsequent research to focus on optimizing speech-processing strategies. Early implant designs had problems with interaction between electrodes with synchronous electrode firing causing poor speech discrimination and even uncomfortable loudness summation. Continuous interleaved sampling was therefore introduced, which improved the performance by stimulating adjacent electrodes at fractionally different times at a small cost to temporal resolution. This concept has been taken one step further by pairing distant electrodes (e.g., 1, 5, 2, and 6, etc.) to avoid current summation, although so far results have been disappointing.

Feature extraction strategies attempt to extract the most important features of the signal. Initially, strategies filtered speech according to formants (F0/F1/F2), but this approach led to the loss of high-frequency resolution, which is required for consonant recognition. To overcome this, new coding strategies such as MPEAK were introduced in the late 1980s, which transmitted more high frequency information. SPEAK was then introduced in the 1990s using 20 bandpass filters and 20 envelope detectors. Rather than sending all 20 envelopes to the electrodes, 5–10 selected critical envelopes were used, as per the "n of M" strategies, which select *n* maxima from a total of *m* processing bands for stimulation.

Research continues to target improved performance in speech recognition, listening to music, speech perception in multi-talker babble or background noise and better sound localization. These goals may eventually be realized by maximizing the fine structure information encoded by speech processors and mimicking normal cochlear function as closely as possible.

Current Developments in Cochlear Implant Design

Although there have been gradual improvements in sound processing strategies, in recent years, most progress has been made with implant hardware including improvements in the electrode array, microphone and batteries. The primary objectives of these developments have been to optimize the interface between electrode and cochlear nerve and to optimize and even improve the health of the cochlea and cochlear nerve. Advancements are also taking place to optimize the convenience of being an implant recipient, for example, through the development of fully implantable devices, MRI compatible devices and devices that can be remotely programmed. Manufacturers attempt to make each new generation of device more robust with greater long-term reliability, more energy efficiency and crucially with decreased user performance variance.

Optimizing the Electrode/Neural Interface and Controlling the Current Spread

Current problems with electrode arrays include poor spatial selectivity, insertional trauma and high power consumption. A number of modifications to current electrode designs have been made in an attempt to overcome these, including pre-curved electrode arrays to allow better proximity between electrode and neuron as well as thin and flexible electrodes to reduce insertional trauma. Novel stimulation strategies have also been developed including current steering techniques, optical stimulation and piezoelectric stimulation.

Modiolar Hugging Electrodes

Current spread from electrodes results in poor spatial selectivity. This can be potentially reduced by bringing the electrodes closer to neural structures. A recent study determined electrode-to-modiolus distance in arrays from 3 manufacturers using CT imaging in 137 implanted ears (2,365 electrodes). They found that electrode distance only contributes minimally to the current level required for suprathreshold stimulation. Electrode-to-modiolus distance also does not influence speech scores but greater reductions in distance may reduce the current requirements enough to prolong battery life in an implantable device. In the past, this was achieved with pre-curved, modiolar hugging electrodes, but a recent design with promise is a hydrogel-based actuated electrode shaft which curves when in contact with saline solution mimicking the perilymph. It is unclear whether better access to apical nerve fibres would give improved high-frequency spatial resolution. A randomized controlled trial has, however, showed clear benefit when using a standard (26.4 mm) array over a medium (20.9 mm) array in the early post-activation period.

Intraneural Electrodes

An alternative means by which power requirements could be reduced and spatial resolution improved is the development of intraneural electrodes. These are implanted into the modiolus to bring electrodes in closer proximity with the spiral ganglion cells resulting in their direct stimulation. This may also reduce facial nerve stimulation and allow implantation in patients in whom the cochlea is not implantable. Middlebrooks and Snyder found that they could stimulate spiral ganglion cells with less current by using a straight modiolar electrode array in cats. Widening the round window before making a hole in the osseous spiral lamina allowed array advancement onto the modiolar nerve. Unfortunately, a disadvantage of intraneural electrodes is the increased likelihood of neuronal injury. Arts et al. [3] mitigated against this by using electrodes with thin shanks. The biggest hurdle, however, is the variable spatial arrangement of the tonotopic map within modiolar nerve fibres. Although electrodes can be frequency mapped during programming, the current spread is likely to be an issue. Alternatively, implantation onto the cochlear nerve trunk proximal to the modiolus could be considered although there may, again, be significant difficulties in achieving tonotopic stimulation at this level.

Current Steering

Another method of controlling current spread is by creating virtual electrodes using current steering. This involves activating 2 adjacent electrodes to stimulate neurons in between the electrodes. Alternatively, current focusing uses 2 or more intracochlear electrodes as active electrodes and ground electrodes, allowing narrow regions of spiral ganglion cells to be stimulated [4]. It is worth noting that using current steering and virtual channels relies on a good population of spiral ganglion cells [1, 2]. Benefits from these strategies are currently small and in some patients use of these techniques actually has a detrimental effect, but future developments may lead to greater improvements [5]. Bilateral cochlear implantation theoretically could allow stimulation of the range of the tonotopic map to be shared or staggered across both ears, thereby doubling the distance between stimulation sites within each cochlear thus improving spatial resolution.

Optical Stimulation

Optical, rather than electrical, stimulation may also improve spatial resolution. It relies on the principle that light energy excites certain cells.

this technique is not adequate to power existing cochlear implant technology but may become so in the future.

Speech Processor
Implanting the speech processor is more straightforward, with the main requirement being to ensure it is hermetically sealed and durable. This technology already exists, and has been employed in previous trials of fully implantable devices [3].

Conclusion

Cochlear implant design is likely to continue to evolve rapidly to achieve the audiological, practical and financial goals desired. Developing an affordable, invisible, reliable implant that produces sound quality which matches that of normal hearing individuals is the ultimate goal, although achieving this is a major challenge.

References

1 Krishnamoorthy K, Samy RN, Shoman N: The challenges of starting a cochlear implant programme in a developing country. Curr Opin Otolaryngol Head Neck Surg 2014;22:367–372.
2 Khan M, Mukhtar N, Saeed SR, Ramsden RT: The Pakistan (Lahore) cochlear implant programme: issues relating to implantation in a developing country. J Laryngol Otol 2007;121:745–750.
3 Arts HA, Jones DA, Anderson DJ: Prosthetic stimulation of the auditory system with intraneural electrodes. Ann Otol Rhinol Laryngol Suppl 2003;191:20–25.
4 Wilson BS, Dorman MF: Cochlear implants: current designs and future possibilities. J Rehabil Res Dev 2008;45: 695–730.
5 Friesen LM, Shannon RV, Baskent D, Wang X: Speech recognition in noise as a function of the number of spectral channels: comparison of acoustic hearing and cochlear implants. J Acoust Soc Am 2001;110:1150–1163.
6 Wilson BS, Dorman MF: Cochlear implants: a remarkable past and a brilliant future. Hear Res 2008;242:3–21.
7 Cohen LT, Saunders E, Knight MR, Cowan RS: Psychophysical measures in patients fitted with Contour and straight Nucleus electrode arrays. Hear Res 2006; 212:160–175.
8 Wackym PA, Firszt JB, Gaggl W, Runge-Samuelson CL, Reeder RM, Raulie JC: Electrophysiologic effects of placing cochlear implant electrodes in a perimodiolar position in young children. Laryngoscope 2004;114:71–76.
9 Middlebrooks JC, Snyder RL: Auditory prosthesis with a penetrating nerve array. J Assoc Res Otolaryngol 2007;8: 258–279.
10 Bonham BH, Litvak LM: Current focusing and steering: modeling, physiology, and psychophysics. Hear Res 2008;242: 141–153.
11 Buechner A, Frohne-Buechner C, Stoever T, Gaertner L, Battmer RD, Lenarz T: Comparison of a paired or sequential stimulation paradigm with advanced bionics' high-resolution mode. Otol Neurotol 2005;26:941–947.
12 Tuft BW, Li S, Xu L, Clarke JC, White SP, Guymon BA, et al: Photopolymerized microfeatures for directed spiral ganglion neurite and Schwann cell growth. Biomaterials 2013;34:42–54.
13 Brors D, Bodmer D, Pak K, Aletsee C, Schäfers M, Dazert S, et al: EphA4 provides repulsive signals to developing cochlear ganglion neurites mediated through ephrin-B2 and -B3. J Comp Neurol 2003;462:90–100.
14 Rask-Andersen H, Boström M, Gerdin B, Kinnefors A, Nyberg G, Engstrand T, et al: Regeneration of human auditory nerve. In vitro/in video demonstration of neural progenitor cells in adult human and guinea pig spiral ganglion. Hear Res 2005;203:180–191.
15 Glueckert R, Pfaller K, Kinnefors A, Rask-Andersen H, Schrott-Fischer A: The human spiral ganglion: new insights into ultrastructure, survival rate and implications for cochlear implants. Audiol Neurootol 2005;10:258–273.
16 Littlefield PD, Vujanovic I, Mundi J, Matic AI, Richter CP: Laser stimulation of single auditory nerve fibers. Laryngoscope 2010;120:2071–2082.
17 Hernandez VH, Gehrt A, Reuter K, Jing Z, Jeschke M, Mendoza Schulz A, et al: Optogenetic stimulation of the auditory pathway. J Clin Invest 2014;124:1114–1129.
18 Carland EM, Stoddart PR, Cadusch PJ, Fallon JB, Wade SA: Effect of embedded optical fibres on the mechanical properties of cochlear electrode arrays. Med Eng Phys 2016;38:155–162.
19 Von Békésy G, Wever EG: Experiments in Hearing. New York, McGraw-Hill, 1960.
20 Inaoka T, Shintaku H, Nakagawa T, Kawano S, Ogita H, Sakamoto T, et al: Piezoelectric materials mimic the function of the cochlear sensory epithelium. Proc Natl Acad Sci U S A 2011;108: 18390–18395.
21 Lazard DS, Vincent C, Venail F, Van de Heyning P, Truy E, Sterkers O, et al: Pre-, per- and postoperative factors affecting performance of postlinguistically deaf adults using cochlear implants: a new conceptual model over time. PLoS One 2012;7:e48739.
22 McElveen JT, Cunningham CD: Cochlear implantation in the congenitally malformed ear. Oper Tech Otolayngol Head Neck Surg 2010;21:243–247.

23 Beltrame MA, Birman CS, Escario JC, Kassouma J, Manolidis S, Pringle MB, et al: Common cavity and custom-made electrodes: speech perception and audiological performance of children with common cavity implanted with a custom-made MED-EL electrode. Int J Pediatr Otorhinolaryngol 2013;77:1237–1243.

24 Carlson ML, Neff BA, Link MJ, Lane JI, Watson RE, McGee KP, et al: Magnetic resonance imaging with cochlear implant magnet in place: safety and imaging quality. Otol Neurotol 2015;36:965–971.

25 Wagner F, Wimmer W, Leidolt L, Vischer M, Weder S, Wiest R, et al: Significant artifact reduction at 1.5T and 3T MRI by the use of a cochlear implant with removable magnet: an experimental human cadaver study. PLoS One 2015; 10:e0132483.

Richard Irving
ENT Department, 4th Floor Nuffield House, University Hospital Birmingham
Mindelsohn Way
Edgbaston, Birmingham B15 2TH (UK)
E-Mail Richard.Irving@uhb.nhs.uk

Lloyd SKW, Donnelly NP (eds): Advances in Hearing Rehabilitation.
Adv Otorhinolaryngol. Basel, Karger, 2018, vol 81, pp 114–122 (DOI: 10.1159/000485541)

Pharmacological Issues in Hearing Rehabilitation

Philip A. Bird[a] · Michael J. Bergin[b]

[a]Department of Surgery, University of Otago, and [b]Otolaryngology Head and Neck Surgery Registrar, Christchurch Hospital, Christchurch, New Zealand

Abstract

Surgery aimed at hearing rehabilitation risks damaging residual inner ear function, especially cochlear implant surgery. Pharmacological intervention to reduce this risk has shown great promise in animal models. The challenge is to deliver medication to the appropriate part of the inner ear in appropriate concentrations for long enough to be effective. Barriers to achieving these goals include: the blood/labyrinth barrier, limiting systemic drug delivery to the inner ear, slow rates of diffusion from the base of the cochlea to the apex, limiting intratympanic delivery from the middle ear to the cochlear apex, delayed intracochlear fibrosis, requiring extended medication delivery postoperatively. Intracochlear drug delivery via a drug-eluting cochlear implantation (CI) electrode may solve many of these pharmacologic issues. It is likely that more than one medication will be necessary to maximize inner ear protection and this may include steroids and appropriate growth factors. Such protection may also be helpful for otologic surgical procedures other than CI that have lower risks to hearing.

Introduction

Surgical intervention to rehabilitate hearing function presents risk to residual hearing. Of the available interventions, cochlear implantation (CI) has the greatest risk of losing residual hearing, but all middle ear surgery is associated with a risk of reducing inner ear function.

Whilst changes in surgical technique and refinements of prosthetic devices have reduced the risks, there is great scope for "protection" of the cochlea and vestibular organs with pharmacological intervention. Intervening with pharmaceuticals presents several challenges in delivering the right agent in sufficient concentration to the appropriate part of the inner ear for sufficient time to counteract the negative effects of surgery. These considerations need to be compatible with surgical schedules, patient comfort and safety.

This discussion will focus mainly on the protection of residual hearing in CI. Corticosteroids have been researched more extensively than other drugs, so more is known about their pharmacology, and much of this discussion will concern them. Several other potential agents will also be discussed.

Modes of Delivery to the Inner Ear/Inner Ear Pharmacokinetics

How a drug is delivered to the inner ear must be balanced with its mechanism of action, its pharmacodynamics and the therapeutic target. For example, in CI in patients with residual hearing the issues for the surgeon are reducing fibrosis within the scala tympani and preserving hair cells, supporting cells and spiral ganglion neurons, especially in the apical regions of the cochlea to preserve residual hearing. When considering preserving residual vestibular function, delivery issues may be somewhat different due to the different location of vestibular receptors.

Drugs may be delivered locally or systemically. Systemic delivery has advantages of not interfering with the surgical procedure, the ability to deliver the medication at any time, and more diffuse delivery throughout the cochlea. The disadvantages are firstly subjecting the rest of the body to potential side effects of the drug; and secondly, there are issues with drug delivery across the blood/labyrinth barrier. The blood/labyrinth barrier is created by the endothelial cells lining the strial blood vessels which are sealed by tight junctions, and limit entry of substances delivered systemically into the inner ear. When compared to local administration, systemic drug administration achieves lower concentrations in cochlear perilymph in the basal turn [1, 2], but not necessarily to the apex.

The methods of local administration are transtympanic, intratympanic or intracochlear. Transtympanic refers to an injection across the tympanic membrane, while intratympanic placement occurs during surgery. Drugs delivered transtympanically and intratympanically gain entry via the round and oval windows. The round window membrane is semipermeable and consists of a middle ear-facing layer of cuboidal epithelial cells, and an inner ear-facing layer of mesothelial cells, with a loosely organized connective tissue layer in between. Although the epithelial cells have tight junctions, the round window membrane does not impede the movement of most drugs into the inner ear. Movements may be intercellular or transcellular via pinocytosis, with molecules as large as 1 μm being able to pass through the membrane. While many substances pass through the round window via simple diffusion, the rate of passage varies according to size, electrical charge, lipophilicity and concentration gradients [3]. Recently, inner ear imaging studies after intratympanic gadolinium [4] have shown that significant substance movement occurs across the oval window as well.

Transtympanic and intratympanic drug delivery is simple to perform and relatively inexpensive, but provides variable and short-lived drug entry into the inner ear [5–7]. The drug may be lost down the Eustachian tube or taken up by the middle ear mucosa. Movement across the round and oval windows may be reduced by mucosal disease. The round window niche may be blocked by a mucosal fold or may develop an air bubble which limits drug absorption.

To overcome some of the issues with intratympanic solutions, slow release carriers have been developed. Thermoreversible polaxamer 407 hydrogels may contain substances including dexamethasone [8] or triamcinolone acetylide [9], and provide slow release of the drug over weeks to months. The unique properties of the gel enable it to exist in liquid form at room temperature and then as a gel at body temperature, allowing them to be easily injected and remain in the middle ear cavity. Sustained delivery is possible for up to 3 months [8].

After drug delivery to the middle ear, several factors determine the drug concentration and distribution. The acronym LADME is a useful way of describing inner ear pharmacokinetics. It corresponds to Liberation, Absorption, Distribution, Metabolism, and Elimination. Liberation refers to how much drug is released from the gel or solution. Absorption is influenced by size and polarity of drug molecules. Distribution via diffusion between the scala tympani and scala vestibuli occurs relatively rapidly, but is much slower from the cochlea base to apex. This slow apical movement leads to a significant concentration gradient throughout the length of the scala tympani. For dexamethasone, this factor plus relatively rapid elimination, could mean insignificant drug delivery to the cochlear apex, even with sustained intratympanic delivery [10]. Lipophilic steroid molecules may pass across the round window more effectively than more water soluble molecules.

Another method of delivery which can potentially overcome the shortcomings of the systemic and intratympanic routes, is intracochlear drug delivery. This requires direct penetration of the cochlea and in itself may be traumatic. Delivery may be via slow infusion, drug-eluting cochlear implant arrays or nanoengineered supraparticles. Slow infusion techniques are not a practical solution in the surgical setting. Infusion cannulae associated with the cochlear implant array have been used in animal experiments, but having an extra portal is highly likely to cause infection and should not be used during CI. Cochlear implant arrays can be coated with substances such as hydrogels, silicone-based polymers or polypyrrole which slowly release drugs into the cochlea. There are a number of studies utilizing drug-eluting electrodes in animal models which will be discussed later.

Nanoengineered supraparticles can be assembled using a combination of mesoporous silica and poly-L-glutamic acid and loaded with the drug in question. The materials are biologically safe and can be assembled into large enough particles (100–500 μm) to be easily handled and placed into the scala tympani during surgery [11]. Supraparticles can be engineered to release a number of different drugs, and have been used in experimental models to deliver neurotrophins.

Inner Ear Trauma after Surgery

Cochlear Implantation

Opening the inner ear and inserting a foreign body along the scala tympani, unsurprisingly may lead to a reduction in residual hearing. Steps of the procedure which may cause injury include drilling, hydraulic trauma from a pressure wave during insertion, blood and bone dust entering the scala tympani, direct insertional trauma which may be minor or major with penetration of the basilar membrane and/or the osseous spinal lamina, bacterial infection and finally foreign body reaction to the electrode [12–17]. Major insertional trauma is of course highly unlikely to be modified by medication.

Direct macroscopic trauma leads to necrosis and programmed cell death, not only in the sites of direct trauma but also at more remote sites over time. Later, fibrosis around the electrode may significantly contribute towards loss of residual hearing secondary to effects on cochlear mechanics, independent of inflammatory causes of delayed hearing [18–20, 22]. The later development of fibrosis may well be a major cause of delayed hearing loss which has been reported to occur in up to 30% of people over time, even with 10 mm electrodes [21]. These findings suggest that prevention of fibrosis should be a major goal of pharmacotherapy in CI.

Middle Ear Surgery

Sensorineural hearing loss may also be seen following middle ear surgery, and it is the basal, high frequencies which are most sensitive to this trauma [23]. When only these high frequencies are investigated, a loss may be seen in 4% of ossiculoplasty patients [24], 7% of myringoplasty patients [25], 10% of stapedectomy patients [26], and 18% of mastoidectomy patients [27]. When the extended high frequencies (<20 kHz) are examined, up to a third of stapedectomy patients sustain a measurable loss [28]. This basal region of the cochlea is likely to be more sensitive to trauma because it is at a watershed area between the cochlear artery and the cochlear ramus of the vestibulocochlear artery [29]. Hearing loss may be from physical movement of the ossicular chain, noise, perilymph leak and bleeding into the vestibule. It is unknown where the locus of injury occurs, but hair cells, neuronal components and the stria vascularis are likely sites of trauma, and should therefore be the target of pharmacologic intervention.

Candidate Drugs for Inner Ear Protection

Corticosteroids

Both glucocorticoid and mineralocorticoid receptors are found in the inner ear with significant concentrations of glucocorticoid receptors in the inner and outer hair cells, the spiral ganglion neurons and the spiral ligament [30–33]. It is often assumed that corticosteroids exert an anti-inflammatory effect on the inner ear, but their actions are more complicated than this. Much of the potential benefit of corticosteroids in improving the hearing in conditions such as sudden sensorineural hearing loss and Meniere's disease may actually be due to their effect on mineralocorticoid receptors [34]. Approximately 85% of 17,500 genes in the mouse inner ear are either upregulated or downregulated by a single dose of intratympanic dexamethasone, with a somewhat smaller proportion of gene changes when given systemically [35].

Anti-inflammatory actions of corticosteroids protect against cochlear implant insertion trauma in a number of ways [36]. There is an upregulation of anti-apoptosis genes and downregulation of pro-apoptosis genes. Dexamethasone reduces interleukins, tumor necrosis factor-alpha and other inflammatory cytokines, and also positively influences hair cell protection pathways.

L-N-Acetylcysteine

L-N-Acetylcysteine is a free radical scavenger and a prodrug of cysteine, which is a precursor to the antioxidant glutathione. It provides protection against hydroxyl radicals and lipid peroxidase, and blocks the mitogen activated protein/cJun N-terminal kinase pathway to apoptosis. L-N-acetylcysteine has shown promise in protecting the inner ear from a number of ototoxic medications [37, 38] and from noise-induced hearing loss in animal and human studies [39, 40].

Neurotrophins and Growth Factors

Neurotrophins are peptides such as brain-derived neurotrophin factor and neurotrophin 3, and are essential for normal maintenance and integrity of the hair cell synapse. They are secreted by hair cells and supporting cells. Loss of these cells following cochlear insult results in reduced neurotrophins which then contributes towards spiral ganglion cell degeneration. Administering exogenous neurotrophins reduces spiral ganglion cell degeneration [41]. Neurotrophin administration also leads to the proliferation of spiral ganglion cell dendrites [42, 43]. Both of these effects have the potential to improve preservation of residual hearing and improve cochlear implant performance.

Insulin-like growth factor (IGF-1) is primarily produced in the liver and has multiple effects. It stimulates cell growth, especially in neural tissue, and is an inhibitor of programmed cell death. Hepatocyte growth factor (HGF) is secreted by mesenchymal cells and acts as a multifunctional cytokine on cells, mainly of epithelial origin. Both IGF-1 and HGF have been used in animal experiments to protect hair cells from noise, ototoxic drugs and ischemic injury [44–46].

References

1 Parnes LS, Sun AH, Freeman DJ: Corticosteroid pharmacokinetics in the inner ear fluids: an animal study followed by clinical application. Laryngoscope 1999;109:1–17.

2 Bird PA, Murray DP, Zhang M, Begg EJ: Intratympanic versus intravenous delivery of dexamethasone and dexamethasone sodium phosphate to cochlear perilymph. Otol Neurotol 2011;32:933–936.

3 Goycoolea MV, Lundman L: Round window membrane. Structure function and permeability: A review. Microsc Res Tech 1997;36:201–211.

4 King EB, Salt AN, Eastwood HT, O'Leary SJ: Direct entry of gadolinium into the vestibule following intratympanic applications in Guinea pigs and the influence of cochlear implantation. J Assoc Res Otolaryngol 2011;12:741–751.

5 Plontke SK, Salt AN: Quantitative interpretation of corticosteroid pharmacokinetics in inner ear fluids using computer simulations. Hear Res 2003;182:34–42.

6 Bird PA, Begg EJ, Zhang M, Keast AT, Murray DP, Balkany TJ: Intratympanic versus intravenous delivery of methylprednisolone to cochlear perilymph. Otol Neurotol 2007;28:1124–1130.

7 Plontke SK, Mukulec AA, Salt AN: Rapid clearance of methylprednisolone after intratympanic application in humans. Otol Neurotol 2008a;29:732–733.

8 Piu F, Wang X, Fernandez R, Dellamary L, Harrop A, Ye Q et al: OTO-104: a sustained-release dexamethasone hydrogel for the treatment of otic disorders. Otol Neurotol 2001;32:171–179.

9 Honeder C, Engleder E, Schopper H, Gabor F, Reznicek G, Wagenblast J, Gstoettner W, Arnoldner C: Sustained release of triamcinolone acetonide from an intratympanically applied hydrogel designed for the delivery of high glucocorticoid doses. Audiol Neurotol 2014;19:193–202.

10 Salt AN, Hartsock JJ, Gill RM, Piu F, Plontke SK: Perilymph pharmacokinetics of markers and dexamethasone applied and sampled at the lateral semicircular canal. J Assoc Res Otolaryngol 2012;13:771–783.

11 Tan J, Wang Y, Yip X, Glynn F, Shepherd RK, Caruso F: Nanoporous peptide particles for encapsulating and releasing neurotrophic factors in an animal model of neurodegeneration. Adv Mater 2012;24:3362–3366.

12 Lehnhardt E: Intracochlear placement of cochlear implant electrodes in soft surgery technique. HNO 2003;41:356–359.

13 Cohen NL: Cochlear implant soft surgery: fact or fantasy? Otolaryngol Head Neck Surg 1997;117:214–216.

14 Kiefer J, Gstoettner W, Baumgertner W, Pok SM, Tillein J, Ye Q, et al: Conservation of low-frequency hearing in cochlear implantation. Acta Otolaryngol 2004;124:272–280.

15 Eshraghi AA: Prevention of cochlear implant electrode damage. Curr Opin Otolaryngol Head Neck Surg 2006;14:323–328.

16 Postelmans JT, van Spronsen E, Grolman W, Stokroos RJ, Tange RA, Mare JM, et al: An evaluation of preservation of residual hearing using the suprameatal approach for cochlear implantation: can this implantation technique be used for preservation of residual hearing? Laryngoscope 2001;121:1794–1799.

17 Bas E, Gupta C, Van de Water TR: A novel organ of corti explant model for the study of cochlear implantation trauma. Anat Rec 2012b;295:1944–1956.

18 Choi CH, Oghalai JS: Predicting the effect of post-implant cochlear fibrosis on residual hearing. Hear Res 2005;205:193–200.

19 Kiefer J, Bohnke F, Adunka O, Arnold W: Representation of acoustic signals in the human cochlea in presence of a cochlear implant electrode. Hear Res 2006;221:36–43.

20 O'Leary SJ, Monksfield P, Kel G, Connolly T, Souter MA, Chang A, Marovic P, O'Leary JS, Richardson R, Eastwood H: Relations between cochlear histopathology and hearing loss in experimental cochlear implantation. Hear Res 2013;298:27–35.

21 Gantz MJ, Hansen MR, Turner CW, Oleson JJ, Reiss LA, Parkinson AJ: Hybrid 10 clinical trial: preliminary results. Audiol Neurotol 2009;14(suppl 1):32–38.

22 Quesnel AM, Nakajima HH, Rosowski JJ, Hansen MR, Gantz BK, Nadol JB Jr: Delayed loss of hearing after hearing preservation cochlear implantation: human temporal bone pathology and implications for etiology. Hear Res 2016;333:225–234.

23 Domenech J, Carulla M: High-frequency audiometric changes after stapedectomy. Scand Audiol Suppl 1988;30:233–235.

24 Schumerber S, Troussier J, Dumas G, Lavieille JP, Nguyen D: Hearing results with the titanium ossicular replacement prostheses. Eur Arch Otorhinolaryngol 2006;263:347–354.

25 de Zinis LO, Cottelli M, Koka M: Inner ear function following underlay myringoplasty. Audiol Neurotol 2010;15:149–154.

26 Sedwick JD, Louden CL, Shelton C: Stapedectomy vs stapedotomy: do you really need a laser? Arch Otolaryngol Head Neck Surg 1997;123:177–180.

27 Ragheb SM, Gantz BJ, Mccabe BF: Hearing results after cholesteatoma surgery: The Iowa experience. Laryngoscope 1987;97:1254–1263.

28 Bird P, Babbage M, O'Beirne G, Bergin M, Macassey E: Patterns of Ultra High-Frequency Hearing Loss Following Stapedectomy. Otology Jubilee 2014 150 Years of the Archiv für Ohrenheilkunde, Halle, Germany, May 2014.

29 Crowe S, Guild S, Polvolgt L: Observations on pathology of high-tone deafness. Bull Johns Hopkins Hosp 1934;54:315–379.

30 Rarey KE, Curtis LM, ten Cate WJ: Tissue specific levels of glucocorticoid receptor within the rat inner ear. Hear Res 1993;64:205–210.

31 Ten Cate WJ, Curtis LM, Small GM, Rarey KE: Localization of glucocorticoid receptors and glucocorticoid receptor mRNAs in the rat cochlea. Laryngoscope 1993;103:865–871.

32 Shimazaki T, Ichimiya I, Suzuki M, Mogi G: Localization of glucocorticoid receptors in the murine inner ear. Ann Otol Rhinol Laryngol 2002;111:1133–1138.

33 Tahera Y, Meltser I, Johansson P, Bian Z, Stierna P, Hansson AC, Canlon B: NF-kappaB mediated glucocorticoid response in the inner ear after acoustic trauma. J Neurosci Res 2006a;83:1066–1076.

34 MacArthur C, Hausman F, Kempton B, Trune DR: Intratympanic steroid treatments may improve hearing via ion homeostasis alterations and not immune suppression. Otol Neurotol 2015;36:1089–1095.

35 Trune D, Delaney K, Hausman F, Kempton B, MacArthur C, Choi D: Transtympanically Delivered Steroids Impact Thousands of Inner Ear Genes of Conventional Systemic Delivery. San Diego, CA, Association Research Otolaryngology, 2012.

36 Eshraghi AA, Dinh CT, Bohorquez J, Angeli S, Abi-Hachem R, Van De Water TR: Local drug delivery to conserve hearing: mechanisms of action of eluted dexamethasone within the cochlea. Cochlear Implants Int 2011;12:S51–S53.

37 Kranzer K, Elamin WF, Cox H, Seddon JA, Ford N, Drobniewski F: A systematic review and meta-analysis of the efficacy and safety of N-acetylcysteine in preventing aminoglycoside-induced ototoxicity: implications for the treatment of multidrug-resistant TB. Thorax 2015;70:1070–1077.

38 Mohan S, Smyth BJ, Namin A, Phillips G, Gratton MA: Targeted amelioration of cisplatin-induced ototoxicity in guinea pigs. Otolaryngol Head Neck Surg 2014;151:836–839.

39 Choi CH, Du X, Floyd RA, Kopke RD: Therapeutic effects of orally administrated antioxidant drugs on acute noise-induced hearing loss. Free Radic Res 2014;48:264–272.

40 Kopke R, Slade MD, Jackson R, Hammill T, Fausti S, Lonsbury-Martin B, Sanderson A, Dreisbach L, Rabinowitz P, Torre P 3rd, Balough B: Efficacy and safety of N-acetylcysteine in prevention of noise induced hearing loss: a randomized clinical trial. Hear Res 2015;323:40–50.

41 Wise AK, Fallon JB, Neil AJ, Pettingill LN, Geaney MS, Skinner SJ, Shepherd RK: Combining cell-based therapies and neural prostheses to promote neural survival. Neurotherapeutics 2011;8:774–787.

42 Wise AK, Richardson R, Hardman J, Clark G, O'Leary S: Resprouting and survival of guinea pig cochlear neurons in response to the administration of the neurotrophins brain-derived neurotrophic factor and neurotrophin-3. J Comp Neurol 2005;487:147–165.

43 Leake PA, Hradek GT, Hetherington AM, Stakhovskaya O: Brain-derived neurotrophic factor promotes cochlear spinal ganglion cell survival and function in deafened developing cats. J Comp Neurol 2011;519:1526–1545.

44 Inaoka T, Nakagawa T, Kikkawa YS, Tabata Y, Ono K, Yoshida M, Tsubouchi H, Ido A, Ito J: Local application of hepatocyte growth factor using gelatin hydrogels attenuates noise-induced hearing loss in guinea pigs. Acta Otolaryngol 2009;129:453–457.

45 Kikkawa YS, Nakagawa T, Tsubouchi H, Ido A, Inaoka T, Ono K, Ito J: Hepatocyte growth factor protects auditory hair cells from aminoglycosides. Laryngoscope 2009;1:2027–2031.

46 Fujiwara T, Hato N, Nakagawa T, Tabata Y, Yoshida T, Kimobuchi H, Takeda S, Hyodo J, Hakuba N, Gyo K: Insulin-like growth factor 1 treatment via hydrogels rescues cochlear hair cells from ischaemic injury. Neuroreport 2008;19:1585–1588.

47 Infante EB, Channer GA, Telischi FF, C, Dinh JT, Vu L, Eshraghi AA, Van De Water TR: Mannitol protects hair cells against tumour necrosis factor a-induced loss. Otol Neurotol 2012;33:1656–1663.

48 Wood JW, Bas E, Gupta C, Selman Y, Eshraghi A, Telischi FF, Van De Water TR: Otoprotective properties of mannitol against gentamicin induced hair cell loss. Otol Neurotol 2014;35:e187–e194.

49 Eshraghi AA, Boel J, Shaikh N, Telischi FF, Bauer B, Guardiola M, Bas E, Van De Water T, Rivera I, Mittal J: A novel combination of drug therapy to protect residual hearing post cochlear implant surgery. Acta Otolaryngol 2016;136:420–424.

50 Honeder C, Landegger LD, Engleder E, Gabor F, Plasenzotti R, Plenk H, et al: Effects of intraoperatively applied glucocorticoid hydrogels on residual hearing and foreign body reaction in a guinea pig model of cochlear implantation. Acta Otolaryngol 2015;135:313–319.

51 Vivero RJ, Joseph DE, Angeli S, He J, Chen S, Eshraghi AA, et al: Dexamethasone base conserves hearing from electrode trauma-induced hearing loss. Laryngoscope 2008;118:2028–2035.

52 Hutten M, Dhanasingh A, Hessler R, Stover T, Esesr KH, Moller M, et al: In vitro and in vivo evaluation of a hydrogel reservoir as a continuous drug delivery system for inner ear treatment. PLoS One 2014;9:e104564.

53 Liu Y, Jolly C, Braun S, Janssen T, Scherer E, Steinhoff J, et al: Effects of dexamethasone-releasing implant on cochleae: a functional, morphological, and pharmacokinetic study. Hear Res 2015;327:89–101.

54 Douchement D, Terranti A, Lamblin J, Salleron J, Siepmann F, Siepmann J, et al: Dexamathasone eluting electrodes for cochlear implantation: effect on residual hearing. Cochlear Implants Int 2015;16:195–200.

55 Stathopoulous D, Chambers S, Enke YL, Timbol G, Risi F, Miller C, et al: Development of a safe dexamethasone-eluting electrode array for cochlear implantation. Cochlear Implants Int 2014;15:254–263.

56 James DP, Eastwood H, Richardson RT, O rsquo Leary SJ: Effects of round window dexamethasone on residual hearing in a guinea pig model of cochlear implantation. Audiol Neurotol 2008;13:86–96.

57 Maini S, Lisnichuk H, Eastwood H, Pinder D, James D, Richardson RT, et al: Targeted therapy of the inner ear. Audiol Neurotol 2009;14:402–410.

58 Chang A, Eastwood H, Sly D, James D, Richardson R, O'Leary S: Factors influencing the efficacy of round window dexamethasone protection of residual hearing post-cochlear implant surgery. Hear Res 2009;255:67–72.

59 Eastwood H, Chang A, Kel G, Sly D, Richardson R, O'Leary SJ: Round window delivery of dexamethasone ameliorates local and remote hearing loss produced by cochlear implantation into the second turn of the guinea pig cochlea. Hear Res 2010;265:25–29.

60 Connolly TM, Eastwood H, Kel G, Lisnichuk H, Richardson R, O'Leary S: Preoperative intravenous dexamethasone prevents auditory threshold shift in a guinea pig model of cochlear implantation. Audiol Neurotol 2011;16:137–144.

61 Quesnel S, Nguyen Y, Elmaleh M, Grayeli AB, Ferrary E, Sterkers O, et al: Effects of systemic administration of methylprednisolone on residual hearing in an animal model of cochlear implantation. Acta Otolaryngol 2011;131:579–584.
62 Kuthubutheen J, Coates H, Rowsell C, Nedzelski J, Chen JM, Lin V: The role of extended preoperative steroids in hearing preservation cochlear implantation. Hear Res 2015;327:257–264.
63 Bas E, Bohorquez J, Goncalves S, Perez E, Dinh CT, Garnham C, Hessler R, Eshraghi AA, Van De Water TR: Electrode array-eluted dexamethasone protects against electrode insertion trauma induced hearing and hair cell losses, damage to neural elements, increases in impedance and fibrosis: a dose response study. Hear Res 2016;337:12–24.
64 Kikkawa YS, Nakagawa T, Ying L, Tabata Y, Tsubouchi H, Ido A, Ito J: Growth factor-eluting cochlear implant electrode: impact on residual auditory function, insertional trauma, and fibrosis. J Transl Med 2014;12:280.
65 Richardson RT, Wise AK, Thompson BC, Flynn BO, Atkinson PJ, Fretwell NJ, Fallon JB, Wallace GG, Shepherd RK, Clark GM, O'Leary SJ: Polypyrrole-coated electrodes for the delivery of charge and neurotrophins to cochlear neurons. Biomaterials 2009;30:2614–2624.
66 Enticott JC, Eastwood HT, Briggs, RJ, Dowell RC, O'Leary SJ: Methylprednisolone applied directly to the round window reduces dizziness after cochlear implantation: a randomised clinical trial. Audiol Neurotol 2011;16:289–303.
67 Rajan GP, Kuthubutheen J, Hedne N, Krishnaswamy J: The role of preoperative, intratympanic glucocorticoids for hearing preservation in cochlear implantation: a prospective clinical study. The Laryngoscope 2012;122:190–195.
68 Sweeney AD, Carlson ML, Zuniga MG, Bennett ML, et al: Impact of perioperative oral steroid use on low-frequency. Otol Neurotol 2015;36:1480–1485.
69 Milewski C, Dornhoffer J, DeMeester C: Possibilities for preserving hearing in labyrinth fistulas of different degrees of severity. Laryngorhinootologie 1995;74:408–412.
70 Riechelmann H, Tholen M, Keck T, Rettinger G: Perioperative glucocorticoid treatment does not influence early post-laser stapedotomy hearing thresholds. Am J Otol 2000;21:809–812.
71 Bagger-Sjöbäck D, Strömbäck K, Hakizimana P, Plue J, Larsson C, Hultcrantz M, Papatziamos G, Smeds H, Danckwardt-Lilleström N, Hellström S, Johansson A, Tideholm B, Fridberger A: A randomised, double blind trial of N-acetylcysteine for hearing protection during stapes surgery. PLoS One 2015;10:e0115657.

Philip A. Bird
Department of Surgery, University of Otago
Level 2, 9 Caledonian Road
Edgeware, Christchurch 8014 (New Zealand)
E-Mail phil.bird@chchorl.co.nz

Lloyd SKW, Donnelly NP (eds): Advances in Hearing Rehabilitation.
Adv Otorhinolaryngol. Basel, Karger, 2018, vol 81, pp 123–132 (DOI: 10.1159/000485577)

Intraoperative Auditory System Monitoring

Hidemi Miyazaki[a] • Per Caye-Thomasen[b, c]

[a]Department of Oto-Rhino-Laryngology, Tokyo Women's Medical University Medical Center East, Tokyo, Japan; [b]Department of Oto-Rhino-Laryngology, Head and Neck Surgery, and Audiology F2074, Copenhagen University Hospital Rigshospitalet and [c]Faculty of Health and Medical Sciences, University of Copenhagen, Copenhagen, Denmark

Abstract

A new electrophysiological system for intraoperative, continuous, near-real time monitoring of cochlear nerve function through acoustic stimulation in the ear canal and recording of the evoked dorsal cochlear nucleus potentials (DNAPs) by a specially designed DNAP electrode placed directly on the brainstem is described. The system is denominated "(cerebellopontine angle) CPA Master" and is designed for hearing preservation surgery in the cerebello-pontine angle, through the retro-sigmoid or the retro-labyrinthine approach. As an additional novelty within the field, the system allows intraoperative mapping and thus precise localization of the cochlear nerve in its entire trajectory from the brainstem to the fundus of the internal auditory canal, which is a major advance in relation to atraumatic dissection of the nerve. The system can be used for surgery of all types of CPA tumors, for example, vestibular schwannomas, meningiomas and epidermoid cysts, but also for vestibular nerve section and vascular decompression. The system also allows evaluation of the electrical functionality of an anatomically intact cochlear nerve in translabyrinthine surgery, thus predicting the benefit of optional cochlear implantation.

Introduction

Electrophysiological auditory response techniques have been used for decades in audiology, otology and neurotology, primarily as diagnostic tools [1, 2]. Auditory brain stem response (ABR), auditory steady state response, otoacoustic emissions and electrocochleography (ECOG) are the most prominent examples. Whereas the use of ABR and electrocochleography to a large extent have been substituted by improved methods of imaging in adult cases of asymmetric hearing loss and suspicion of endolymphatic hydrops (Meniere's disease), all of the above responses/methods are still used extensively in pediatric cases.

Electrophysiological monitoring of auditory function during surgery has gained leverage during recent years. In cochlear implantation of patients with residual hearing, cochlear function can be monitored through electrical stimulation and continuous recording of cochlear responses. This has increased the knowledge of surgical events detrimental to cochlear function and thus

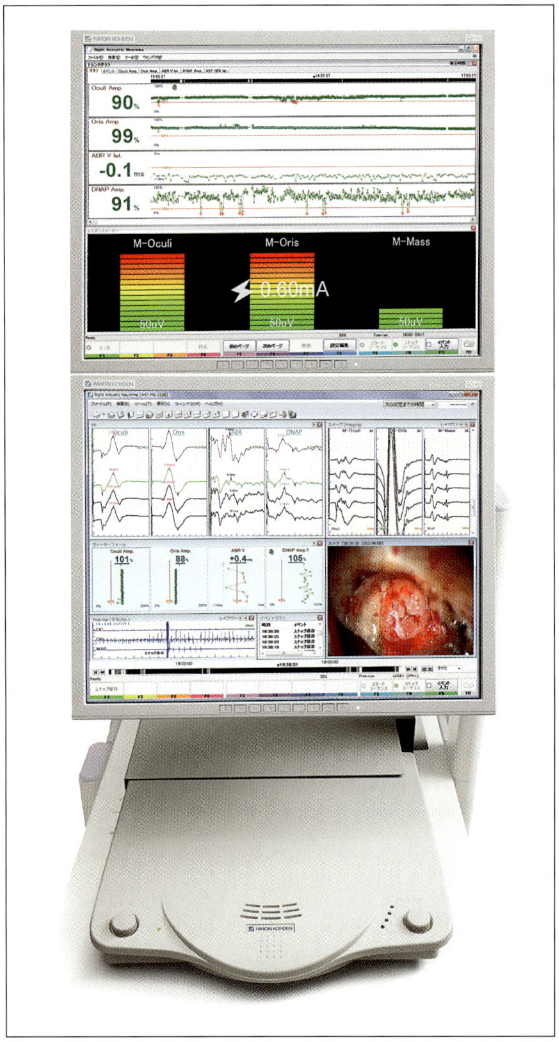

Fig. 1. CPA Master system (NIHONKOHDEN Neuromaster MEE-1000A).

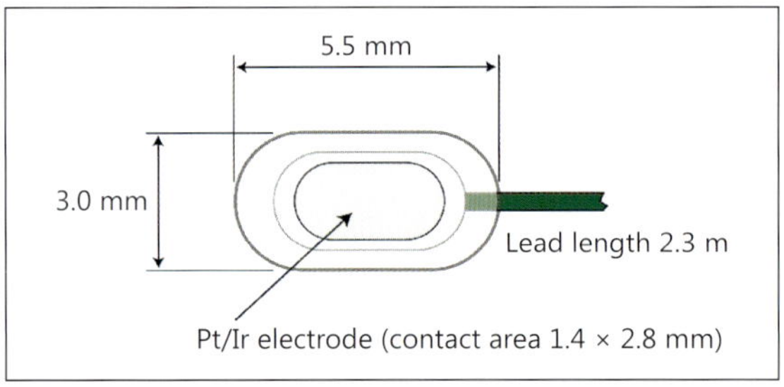

Fig. 2. DNAP electrode.

increased the likelihood of preserved function by the adaptation of atraumatic surgical techniques. Similarly, intraoperative monitoring of auditory function can be used during hearing preservation surgery of vestibular schwannomas. Upon acoustic stimulation in the external ear canal, ABRs are recorded from skin electrodes. A recording delay of up to 1 min has, however, been the primary reason for the abandonment of this method by many surgeons, as a surgical dissection maneuver or event leading to cochlear nerve damage will already have taken place when the system actually detects that damage has occurred. This delay occurs because repetitive testing is needed to achieve a good quality, reliable response. The lack of real time or near-real time feedback on cochlear nerve function is thus a major problem with this monitoring modality, as it does not allow immediate adaptation of the surgical technique to avoid functional damage. Cochlear nerve action potential (CNAP) recording involves the placement of an electrode on the root of the cochlea-vestibular nerve bundle. This can be difficult or even impossible in large tumor cases, and the electrode may easily be displaced during surgical dissection. However, a new device (the cerebellopontine angle [CPA] Master; Fig. 1) offers the possibility of continuously monitoring the cochlear nerve in near-real time using the dorsal cochlear nucleus action potential (DNAP) recorded by placing an electrode (Fig. 2) directly on the dorsal cochlear nucleus (DCN) in the brain stem, via the foramen of Luschka [3]. In addition to the near-real time feedback, the system has another unique feature that allows intraoperative mapping and thus precise localization of the cochlear nerve. This is a major advance in relation to atraumatic dissection of the nerve. This chapter will focus on this new development, which also includes continuous, active monitoring of facial nerve function through an electrode placed on the brain stem, at the facial nerve root exit zone [3].

Hearing Preservation Surgery for Acoustic Tumors (Vestibular Schwannomas)

Surgical approaches for acoustic tumors are broadly divided into approaches intending preservation of hearing and approaches not intending preservation of hearing. Hearing may be preserved by the middle fossa approach, the retrosigmoid approach (RSA) and the retro-labyrinthine approach (RLA), whereas the translabyrinthine approach (TLA) leads to a dead ear. Thus, the TLA is usually chosen when it is not worthwhile preserving the hearing. The fact that there are several approaches aimed at hearing preservation reflects both the difficulty in achieving this goal and the ingenuity of surgeons over time. Details of the various approaches can be found elsewhere in the literature and are not within the scope of this chapter. The relevant main points of the 2 hearing preservation approaches that allow placement of electrodes on the brainstem and thus the use of the new neuromonitoring system will be outlined.

Continuous Monitoring of Nerve Function and Temporary Nerve Stimulation (Mapping) during Surgery

In surgery aimed at preservation of neurological function, both monitoring of nerve function and mapping of the nerve to allow precise localization have important roles. Temporary electrical stimulation to obtain an evoked electromyogram of facial muscle contraction is the most prevalent and pervasive technique for monitoring of facial nerve function. However, this is not monitoring in the true sense of the word, as monitoring should be continuous. Therefore, the technique that temporarily stimulates the facial nerve by electricity is more accurately referred to as facial nerve mapping or localization, in distinction to monitoring. Publications and research reports on continuous monitoring of the facial nerve do exist. However, electrodes need to be positioned intracranially. The new monitoring system presented here includes a facial nerve electrode to be placed directly on the facial nerve root exit zone during surgery. Every 3 s an electrical stimulus is applied to the electrode and the resulting facial muscle contraction is monitored, allowing near-real time monitoring of not only function, but also the level of function during the surgical procedure, as compared to initial baseline measurements. As this book and chapter focuses on hearing function, elaboration on the facial nerve monitoring modality will be reserved for later publications.

Concerning cochlear nerve function, optimal continuous monitoring and mapping techniques have been explored for a number of years and a wide variety of studies have been reported accordingly. Monitoring should be sensitive and stable, and mapping should be accurate, for precise localization of the cochlear nerve. Auditory brainstem response (ABR) has been the most prevalent technique for intraoperative monitoring of cochlear nerve function in acoustic tumor surgery. However, ABR does not allow mapping and thus localization of the cochlear nerve during surgery and as noted above, the recording delay does not allow the desired, near-real time feedback and assessment of function. These features are, however, provided by the CPA Master system, which includes an electrode developed for measuring DNAPs directly on the brainstem.

Near-Real-Time, Continuous Monitoring of Cochlear Nerve Function by DNAP Recording during Surgery

As noted earlier, ABR lacks real-time measurement and mapping capability. In addition, when the hearing is relatively poor (often the case in acoustic tumors), the evoked wave V has a low amplitude, low reproducibility and can be difficult to detect. ABR may, therefore, be considered

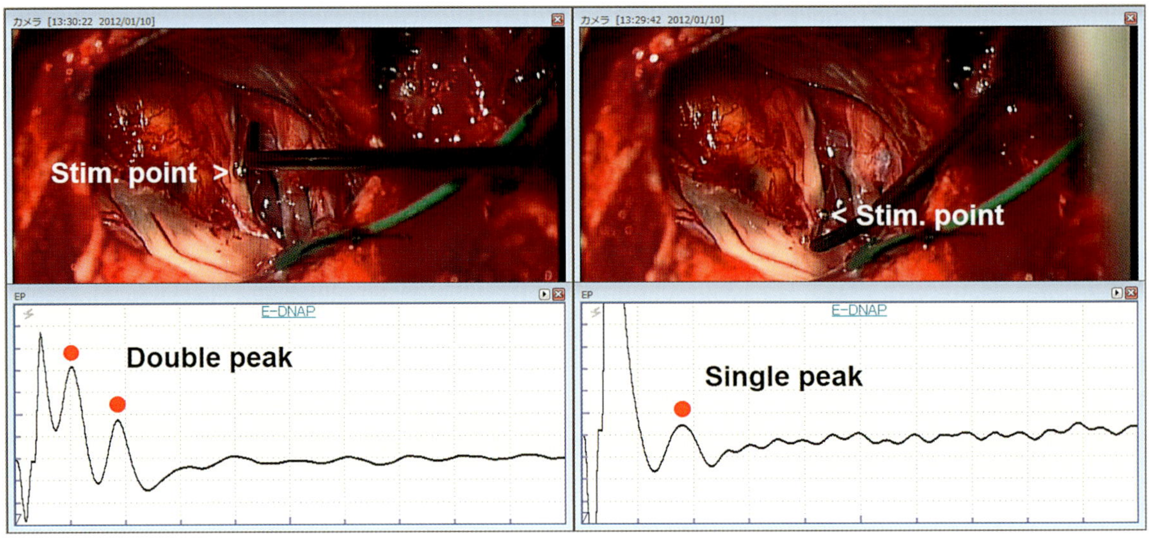

Fig. 3. Cochlear nerve mapping.

as an insufficient or suboptimal tool for intraoperative monitoring.

The use of an electrode placed on the cochlear nerve for measurement of CNAPs has been reported by several centers. Since CNAPs are of high amplitude this method is sensitive. However, the electrode cannot be placed when the cochlear nerve root cannot be identified in the operative field. In addition, measurements are likely to be unstable as it is difficult to fix the electrode in place, and the electrode is therefore frequently displaced during surgery.

The CPA Master system includes a DNAP electrode for measuring action potentials from the DCN in the brainstem, and it was developed to overcome the disadvantages associated with ABR and CNAP monitoring. DNAPs obtained from the DCN are considered to have complex waveforms corresponding to the III–V waves of ABR. The amplitude of DNAP is 10–50 times that of ABR. Therefore, averaging of only 50–200 measurements is sufficient. Thus, DNAP measurement time is 3–12 s, which allows near-real time detection of damage to the cochlear nerve during surgery. Usually, it takes 6 s if the patient has slight hearing loss.

Cochlear Nerve Mapping during Surgery

Another important feature of the CPA Master system is cochlear nerve mapping. The superior olivary nucleus is located upstream from the cochlear nucleus in the brainstem, whereas the nerve cells in the vestibular brainstem nucleus do not synapse in a nucleus upstream. Thus, when weak monopolar electrical stimulation is applied to the 8th cranial nerve (using the same stimulation probe as for facial nerve stimulation), stimulation on the cochlear part of the nerve (electrical DNAP) will evoke 2 action potentials, displayed as double peaks on the monitor screen (the first from the cochlear brainstem nucleus and with around 1 ms delay and the second from the superior olivary nucleus), whereas stimulation on the vestibular part of the nerve only generates one action potential, leading to a single or no peak (Fig. 3). Thus, both vestibular and cochlear fibers can be identified by electrical probe stimulation. The entire trajectory of the cochlear nerve – from the root at the brainstem to the lateral part in the fundus of the internal auditory canal – can be located precisely by stimulation, which is of major importance during nerve/tumor dissection.

In addition, electrical stimulation can be applied by the probe to the cochlea (e.g., on the promontory or the round window), for example, at the end of surgery in case of anatomical, but not functional preservation (by acoustic ear canal stimulus) of the cochlear nerve. The cochlear nerve has preserved its electrical function if a DNAP at the brainstem is elicited by electrical stimulation of the cochlea, indicating that a cochlear implant is an option likely to benefit the patient.

The electrical DNAP requires 50–100 times signal averaging using 0.1–0.4 mA stimulation at 30 Hz. In other words, the surgeon needs to keep the stimulating probe in the same position for about 3 s for accurate measurement.

DNAP Electrode Placement in the Retro-Sigmoid Approach

Monitoring of DNAP requires placement of the DNAP electrode on the brainstem, and this should be done before initiating tumor removal to retrieve initial baseline recordings, which serve as a reference during tumor dissection. Thus, only approaches that allow visualization of the brainstem at the level of the cochlear nuclei before tumor removal are appropriate for DNAP monitoring, that is, the RSA and the RLA.

The RSA involves a craniotomy behind the sigmoid sinus, and although the size of the craniotomy may be varied according to the size of the tumor, the craniotomy size is not important for DNAP electrode placement on the brainstem. The site is, however, important, as a relatively inferior craniotomy allows easy access to the main anatomical landmark, the glossopharyngeal nerve. After identification of the lower cranial nerves, the electrode is inserted into the foramen of Luschka adjacent to the glossopharyngeal nerve, using the anatomical landmarks illustrated in Figure 4. This placement method has the following 2 advantages. First, the electrode is fixed and unlikely to be displaced since the foramen of Luschka is not widely open. Second, dissection and removal of a CPA tumor are not hampered by the electrode, as the cable trajectory is along the glossopharyngeal nerve and further outwards along the inferior edge of the craniotomy. With a low craniotomy, the microscope can be angled in a cranio-caudal direction, allowing excellent lower cranial nerve overview. Then, the arachnoid membrane between the choroid plexus and the glossopharyngeal nerve is dissected, and the electrode is inserted along the nerve so that the electrode faces the glossopharyngeal nerve and eventually comes to sit facing the DCN, as illustrated in Figures 4 and 5. If sufficient DNAPs cannot be obtained, the position of the electrode is adjusted slightly and new measurements are performed. If the foramen of Luschka is opened widely for electrode positioning, it increases the risk of electrode instability. Once DNAPs can be measured stably, the electrode cable is secured by, for example, sutures to the caudal dura mater and the skin inferiorly, so that the electrode cable does not obstruct the operative field and the risk of the drill damaging the cable is minimized. It is also advisable to fix the cable to the sterile drapes with, for example, tape to avoid unexpected pulling.

DNAP Electrode Placement in the Retro-Labyrinthine Approach

After a wide mastoidectomy, the posterior semicircular canal is identified and blue-lined. Bone over the medial and posterior fossa dura, as well as the sigmoid sinus and the jugular bulb is removed [4]. The dura is opened as inferiorly as possible, to allow easy identification of the lower cranial nerves and the choroid plexus (Fig. 6). Care should be taken not to retract the cerebellum. The subsequent steps are as for the RSA. Thus, the arachnoid membrane between the

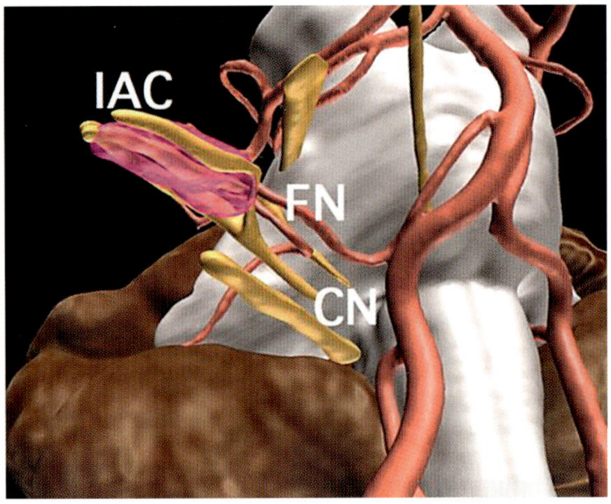

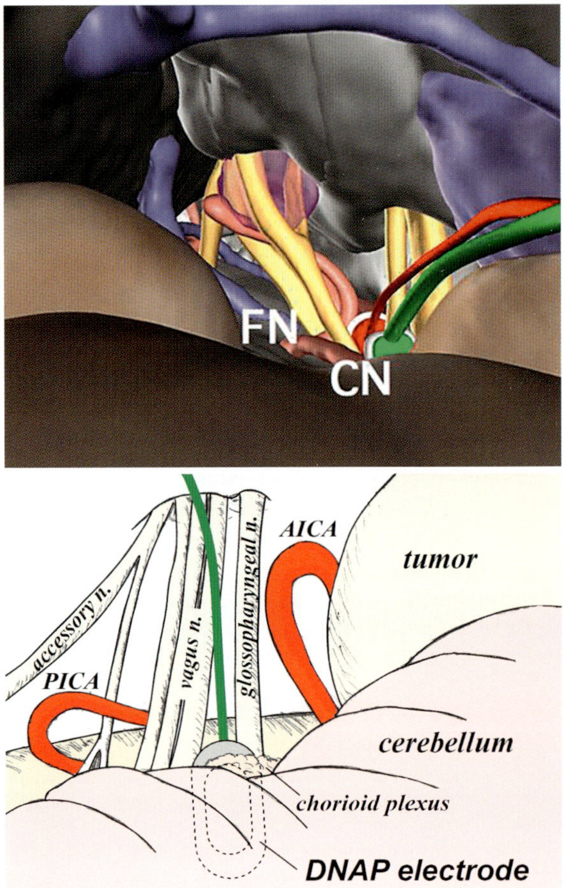

Fig. 4. Drawing demonstrating the anatomy of the CPA relevant to the insertion of the DNAP electrode. The electrode is inserted into the foramen of Luschka along the line of the glossopharyngeal nerve using the choroid plexus as a landmark. Even with small tumors, the DNAP electrode should be placed as soon as possible to allow continuous monitoring before initiating tumor dissection. The initial DNAP measurements will serve as baseline for the remainder of the surgery. If the cerebellum is retracted for a wider operative field, the auditory nerve may be damaged at the root exit zone of the brain stem, which can cause hearing impairment. Brain retraction should, therefore, be minimized. With larger tumors, analysis of the relationship between the foramen of Lushka and the tumor as demonstrated on MRI can help plan the surgery.

choroid plexus and the glossopharyngeal nerve is dissected and the electrode is inserted into the foramen of Luschka along the nerve so that the electrode faces the nerve and eventually comes to sit facing the DCN. The electrode is fixed at the inferior border of the craniotomy as described above, and initial baseline DNAPs are recorded before the dissection of the tumor is commenced. Usually, the electrode can be placed on the brainstem before starting tumor dissection if the extra meatal tumor size is <25 mm. If the lower cranial nerves cannot be identified initially because of a big tumor size or abundant vessels, tumor dissection is initiated and the electrode placed as soon as sufficient access has been created.

Intraoperative Recuperation for Recovery of Cochlear Nerve Function

The goal of continuous monitoring using DNAPs is complete preservation of hearing. To this end, the surgical dissection must be performed without significant functional damage to the cochlear nerve. Cochlear nerve function is monitored by ABR before placement of the DNAP electrode and continuous monitoring is started. A brain retractor should not be used since it may retract or stretch the cochlear nerve, potentially leading to functional damage. DNAP monitoring is started as soon as possible after DNAP electrode placement, and during tumor removal any maneuver causing damage

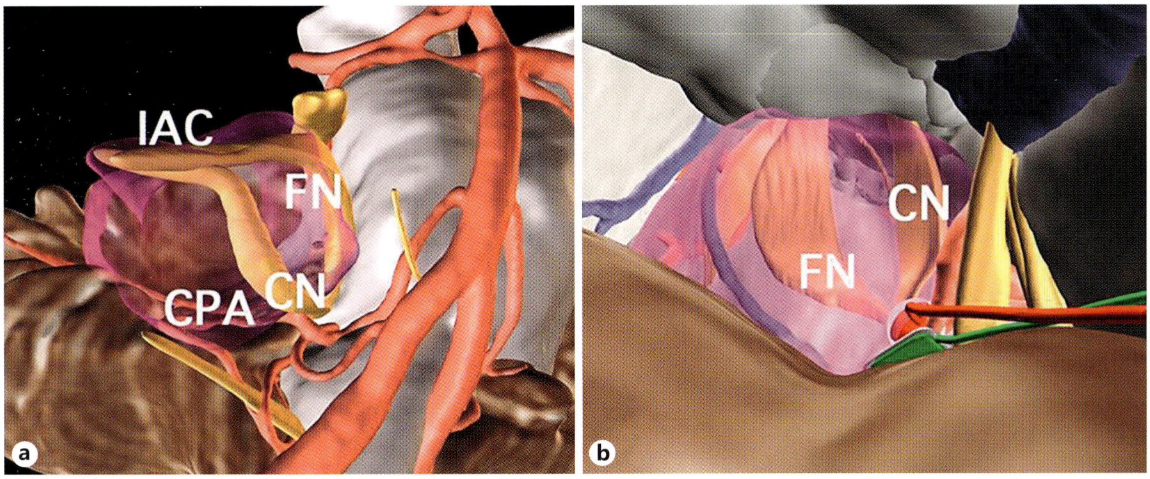

Fig. 5. a, **b** Even in the case of a large tumor, it is still possible to place the DNAP electrode. A key point here is to analyze the positional relation between the lateral recess and the tumor on MRI images. Following localization of the lower cranial nerves and the choroid plexus in the initial phase of surgery, the arachnoid membranes between these can be dissected. For placement on the dorsal cochlear nucleus of the brainstem, the DNAP electrode can then be inserted along the glossopharyngeal nerve into the foramen of Luschka.

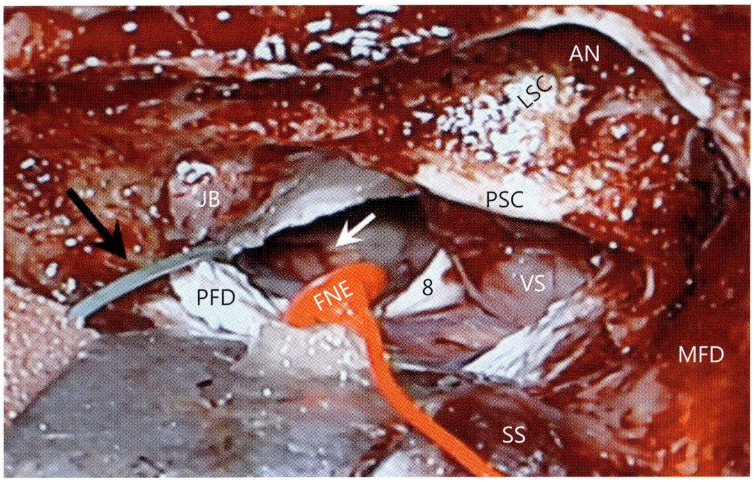

Fig. 6. View through the retro-labyrinthine approach in a patient with a left-sided vestibular schwannoma (VS). The posterior semicircular canal (PSC) has been blue-lined and bone over the middle fossa dura (MFD), the sigmoid sinus (SS), the posterior fossa dura (PFD) and the jugular bulb (JB) has been removed. The PFD has been opened allowing identification of the tumor (VS), the root of the vestibulo-cochlear nerve (8) and the glossopharyngeal nerve (white arrow). The DNAP electrode has been inserted into the foramen of Luschka along the glossopharyngeal nerve and is now fixed on the brainstem, over the dorsal cochlear nucleus. The cable of the DNAP electrode (black arrow) is extending outwards along the inferior edge of the craniotomy, in order not to obstruct tumor dissection. The facial nerve electrode (FNE) is about to be placed at the facial nerve root exit zone on the brainstem. AN, antrum; FNE, facial nerve electrode; JB, jugular bulb; LSC, lateral semicircular canal; MFD, middle fossa dura; PFD, posterior fossa dura; PSC, posterior semicircular canal; SS, sigmoid sinus; VS, vestibular schwannoma; 8, root of 8th cranial nerve.

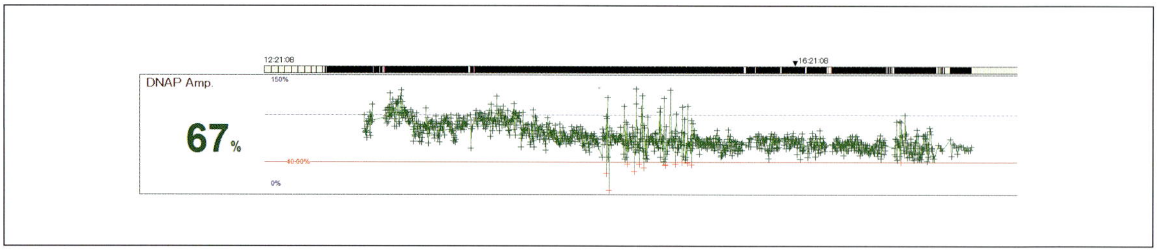

Fig. 7. Monitoring data from a successful case of hearing preservation surgery without any rapid drops in DNAP amplitude during the procedure. Although a mild decrease of amplitude is unavoidable, the hearing class is mostly preserved at preoperative level as long as the final amplitude is 40% or higher, as compared to the initial baseline DNAP measurements.

to the cochlear nerve should be avoided. Functional damage is monitored by change in the DNAP amplitude. With 100% representing the initial baseline amplitude recorded immediately on electrode placement, our preliminary results have shown that final amplitude of at least 40% as compared to baseline is the threshold for hearing preservation. Figure 7 shows a typical DNAP recording with a slow decline in DNAP amplitude over time. The amplitude drop does not, however, reach the critical 40% level. Some decrease in amplitude during the surgical procedure is unavoidable, but if the amplitude drops rapidly, surgery should be paused for at least 15 min and up to an hour to await recovery of the amplitude to at least 40%. This is demonstrated in Figure 5 in which there is a rapid drop in the DNAP amplitude with recovery after pausing the surgery. The degree of recovery is dependent on the degree of injury to the nerve. Recovery (and hence hearing preservation) is, however, unlikely if surgical dissection is continued following a rapid amplitude drop. Thus, even if the surgeon can see an intact nerve, it is important to be guided by the monitoring and pause the dissection when indicated by the functional monitoring. During and after surgery, lessons on dissection maneuvers leading to functional damage of the cochlear nerve can be learned from a coordinated review of the video of the surgery (which is projected on the CPA Master monitoring screen from the microscope) and the DNAP amplitude trend graph (Fig. 7–9). The trend of the graph can thus guide the surgeon, leading to provide an evidence for improved surgical dissection technique, ultimately improving the hearing preservation results.

DNAP Monitoring and Other Indications for CPA Surgery

In all surgical procedures involving the CPA, DNAP monitoring can be helpful to increase the likelihood of hearing preservation. Cochlear nerve mapping is thus a major advantage in vestibular nerve section in patients with refractory Meniere's disease. The technology makes it possible to precisely identify the cochlear and the vestibular part of the 8th cranial nerve bundle, thus ensuring selective and complete section of the vestibular nerve. This reduces not only the risk of hearing impairment, but also the risk of recurrence of attacks of vertigo due to incomplete separation of the vestibular part of the nerve.

DNAP monitoring may also be helpful in surgery for vascular decompression and removal of non-acoustic tumors within the CPA, for example, meningiomas, facial nerve schwannomas, epidermoid and arachnoidal cysts.

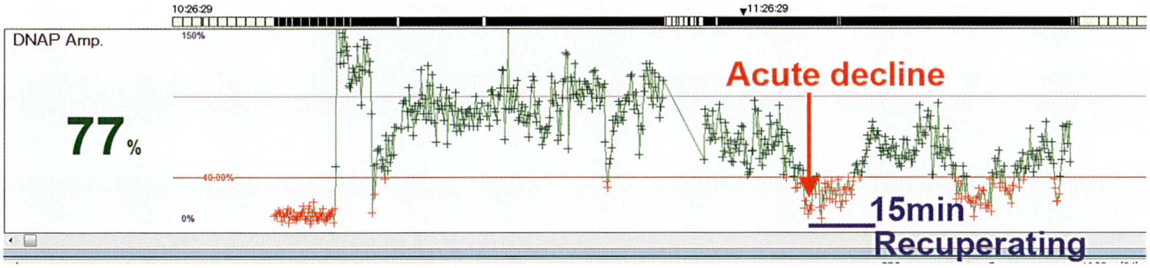

Fig. 8. Monitoring data from a case displaying a rapid drop in DNAP amplitude, followed by recovery after a 15 min pause in dissection. The DNAP monitoring allows recognition of cochlear nerve damage in near-realtime and thus immediate adaptation of the dissection maneuvers, typically leading to pause. Traction is a frequent cause of nerve damage, often recoverable through recuperating treatment. Hearing is typically not preserved if surgery is continued with no pause after the occurrence of a DNAP amplitude decrease.

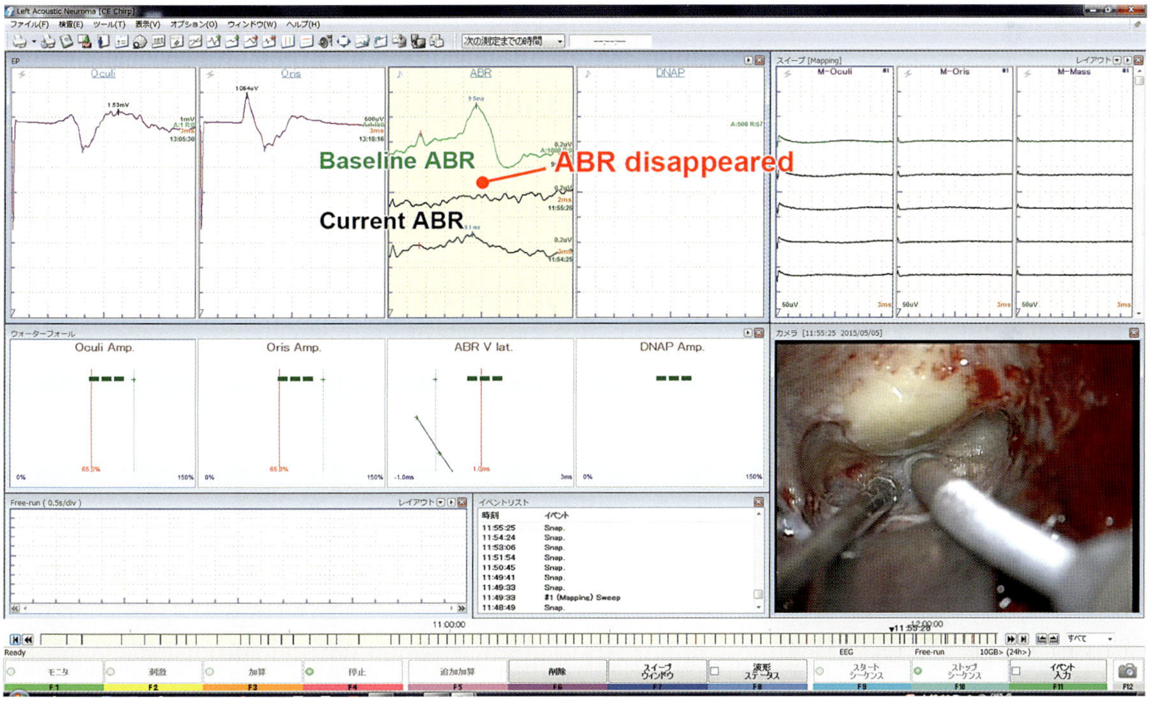

Fig. 9. Monitoring data from a case where ABR rapidly disappeared during drilling around the internal auditory canal in the retro-labyrinthine approach. No DNAPs could be recorded after placement of the DNAP electrode. Cochlear nerve mapping verified cochlear nerve damage, probably due to the heat generated during drilling. In such cases where the cochlear nerve runs on the posterior surface of the tumor, it is often difficult to preserve hearing since surgical dissection has to be performed around the nerve.

Additional Perspectives

Even though acoustic hearing may be lost during attempted hearing preservation surgery to remove a vestibular schwannoma via retrosigmoid or retro-labyrinthine approaches, the cochlear nerve may still be anatomically and electrically intact, thus making the patient a potential candidate for a cochlear implant [5]. If this scenario occurs after a RLA, the CPA Master system allows electrical probe stimulation on the promontory or in the round window niche. Simultaneous recording of DNAPs at the brainstem will clarify whether the cochlear nerve is functional electrically and thus whether the patient will benefit from a subsequent cochlear implantation. This type of cochlear nerve testing is also possible following a TLA, in which acoustic hearing is lost, as long as the integrity of the cochlear nerve is maintained. Again, if electrical cochlear nerve functionality is maintained, cochlear implantation may be possible. This innovation together with increasing evidence for benefit from cochlear implantation in single-sided (acoustic) deafness provides the opportunity for improved hearing rehabilitation in an extended group of patients.

Conclusion

The CPA Master is a new electrophysiological system for intraoperative, continuous, near-real time monitoring of cochlear nerve function through acoustic stimulation in the external ear canal and recording of the evoked DCN potentials (DNAPs) by a specially designed DNAP electrode placed directly on the brainstem. The system is designed for hearing preservation surgery in the cerebello-pontine angle, through the RSA or the RLA. Uniquely, the system also allows intraoperative mapping, and thus precise localization of the cochlear nerve in its entire trajectory from the brainstem to the fundus of the internal auditory canal, which is a major advance in relation to atraumatic dissection of the nerve. The system can be used for surgery of all types of CPA tumors, for example, vestibular schwannomas, meningiomas and epidermoid cysts, but also for vestibular nerve section and vascular decompression. The system also allows the evaluation of the electrical functionality of an anatomically intact cochlear nerve in translabyrinthine surgery, thus predicting benefit from cochlear implantation.

References

1 Miller CA, Brown CJ, Abbas PJ, Chi SL: The clinical application of potentials evoked from the peripheral auditory system. Hear Res 2008;242:184–197.

2 Edwards BM, Kileny PR: Intraoperative neurophysiologic monitoring: indications and techniques for common procedures in otolaryngology-head and neck surgery. Otolaryngol Clin North Am 2005;38:631–642, viii.

3 Nakatomi H, Miyazaki H, Tanaka M, Kin T, Yoshino M, Oyama H, Usui M, Moriyama H, Kojima H, Kaga K, Saito N: Improved preservation of function during acoustic neuroma surgery. J Neurosurg 2015;122:24–33.

4 Russell SM, Roland JT Jr, Golfinos JG: Retrolabyrinthine craniectomy: the unsung hero of skull base surgery. Skull Base 2004;14:63–71.

5 Sanna M, Medina M, Macak A, Rossi G, Sozzi V, Prasad SC: Vestibular schwannoma resection with ipsilateral simultaneous cochlear implantation in patients with normal contralateral hearing. Audiol Neurotol 2016;21:286–295.

Hidemi Miyazaki, MD, PhD
Department of Otorhinolaryngology
Tokyo Women's Medical University Medical Center East
2-1-10 Nishi-ogu, Arakawa-ku
Tokyo 116-8567 (Japan)
E-Mail hidemi.miyazaki@twmu.ac.jp

Lloyd SKW, Donnelly NP (eds): Advances in Hearing Rehabilitation.
Adv Otorhinolaryngol. Basel, Karger, 2018, vol 81, pp 133–145 (DOI: 10.1159/000485579)

Diagnosis and Treatment of Perilymphatic Fistula

Arnaud Deveze[a, b] · Han Matsuda[e] · Maya Elziere[c] · Tetsuo Ikezono[d]

[a]ORL and Skull Base Surgery, Clairval Hospital, Ramsay GDS Health Care, [b]Laboratory of Biomechanism, IFSTTAR UMR T24, Faculty of Medicine Nord, Aix Marseille University, and [c]ORL and Otoneurology Department, European Hospital, Marseille, France; [d]Saitama Medical University Faculty of Medicine, Otorhinolaryngology, [e]Han Matsuda, Saitama Medical University Faculty of Medicine, Otorhinolaryngology, Moroyamamachi, Japan

Abstract

Perilymphatic fistula (PLF) is defined as an abnormal communication between the fluid (perilymph)-filled space of the inner ear and the air-filled space of the middle ear and mastoid, or cranial spaces. PLF is located in the round or oval window, fractured bony labyrinth, microfissures, anomalous footplate, and can occur after head trauma or barotrauma, chronic inflammation, or in otic capsule dehiscence. This clinical entity was initially proposed more than a century ago, yet it has remained a topic of controversy for more than 50 years. The difficulty of making a definitive diagnosis of PLF has caused a long-standing debate regarding its prevalence, natural history, management and even its very existence. In this present study, we will discuss the symptoms, physiological tests (focusing on vestibular assessment) and imaging studies. Referring to a previous criticism, we will share our classification of PLF into 4 categories. Furthermore, we will summarize a nationwide survey using a novel and widely used biomarker (Cochlin-tomoprotein [CTP]) for PLF diagnosis in Japan and present the results of the new diagnostic criteria. PLF is surgically correctable by sealing the fistula, and appropriate recognition and treatment of PLF can improve hearing and balance, and in turn, improve the quality of life of afflicted patients. Therefore, PLF is an especially important treatable disease for otologists.

Introduction

Perilymphatic fistula (PLF) is defined as an abnormal communication between the fluid (perilymph)-filled space of the inner ear and the air-filled space of the middle ear and mastoid, or cranial spaces. PLF may be located in the round or oval window, via a fractured bony labyrinth or via microfissures and may be associated with an anomalous foot plate. They can occur after head trauma, barotrauma, chronic inflammation or in otic capsule dehiscence including stapes surgery.

PLF, as a clinical entity, was initially proposed more than a century ago, yet it has remained a topic of controversy [1]. Patients present with audiovestibular symptoms, but the precise symptoms are variable and often non-specific. It is a

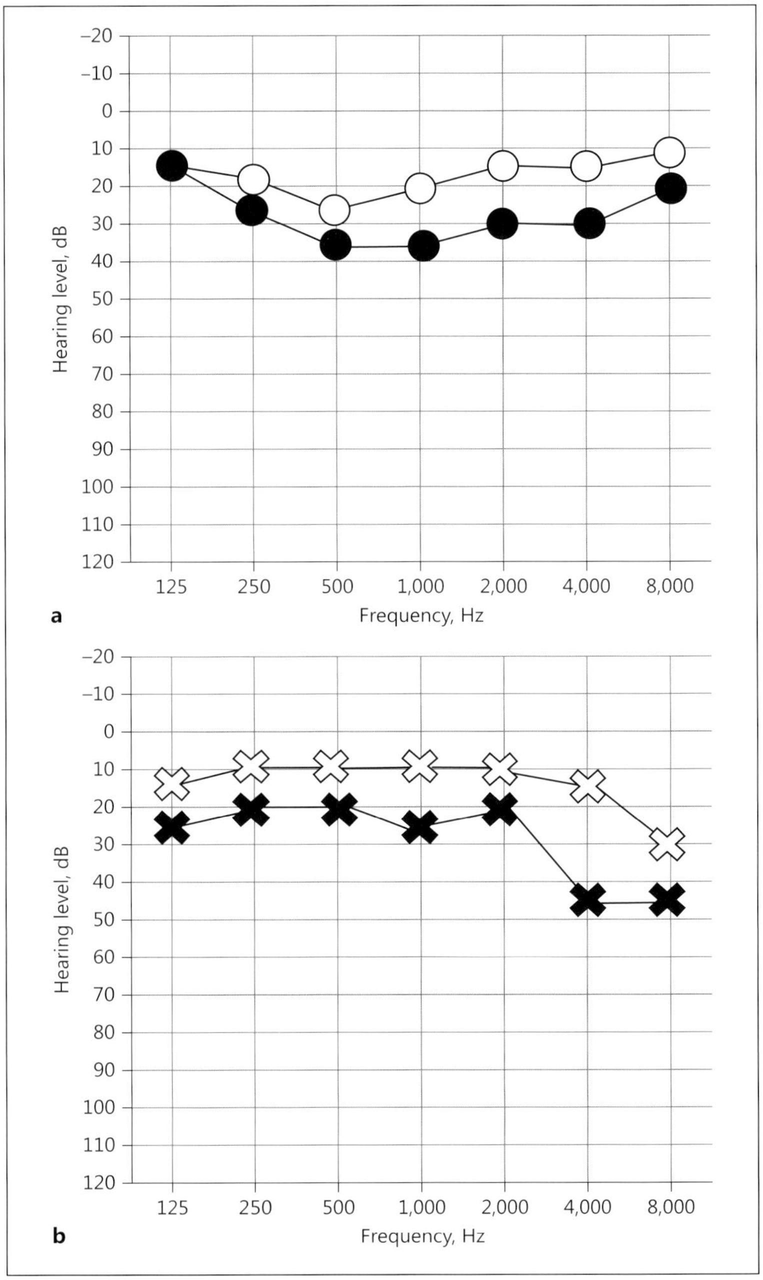

Fig. 1. Two examples of positional audiometry showing a significant decrease in the PTA thresholds when the patient's suspected ear is placed downward for 30 min. Case A (**a**); Case B (**b**).

canal dehiscence, that is, decreased threshold and increased amplitude [19] (Fig. 2b).

Imaging is also an essential part of the diagnosis. Both high resolution CT-scanning and MRI-scanning may be helpful; normal imaging, however, does not exclude a PLF [21]. Apart form the presence of a pneumolabyrinth or an obvious inner ear malformation (both of which are rare but almost pathognomonic) [22], CT imaging may demonstrate liquid filling part or the whole of the

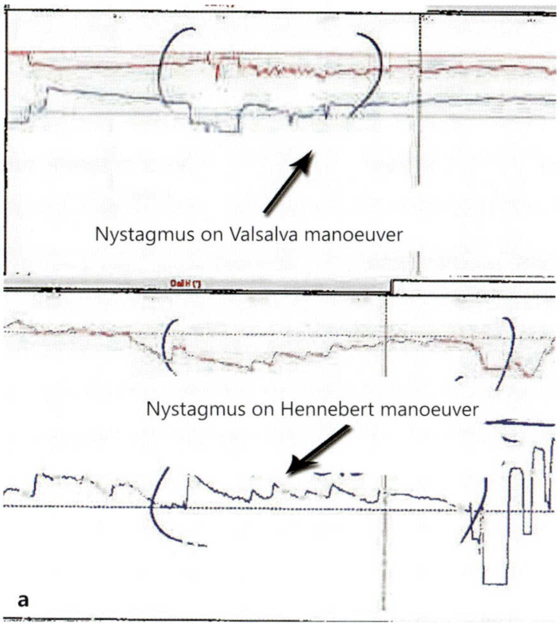

Fig. 2. a Videonystagmography (VNG) showing induced nystagmus on valsalva and Hennebert maneuvers. **b** Cervical vestibular evoked myogenic potentials (cVEMP) suggesting a right-sided PLF. An increase in the amplitude of the wave and decrease in threshold to 80 dB is seen.

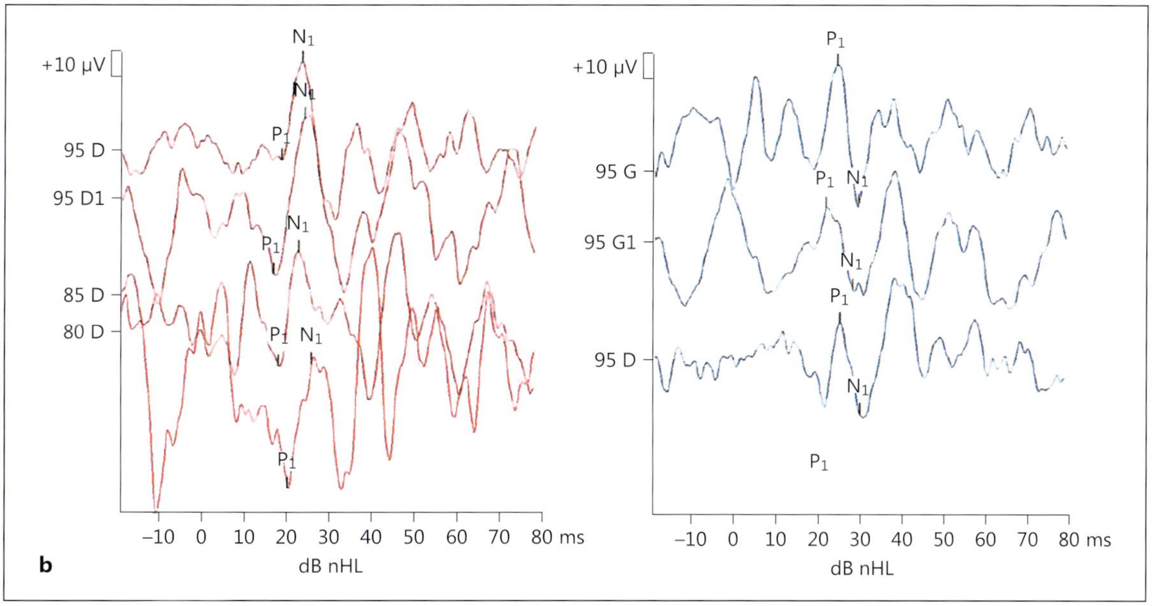

round window niche (presuming the middle ear cleft is well aerated; Fig. 3). With regards to the oval window, the footplate should be carefully evaluated using double-oblique reconstruction to look for luxation, subluxation, blur aspect and the presence of fluid between or around the crura [23]. It is also important to exclude a third window, for example, superior canal dehiscence. MR imaging is mandatory mainly to rule out the differential diagnosis of unilateral cochleo-vestibular symptoms and eliminate a malformation of the inner ear that could be a contributing factor to the development of a PLF.

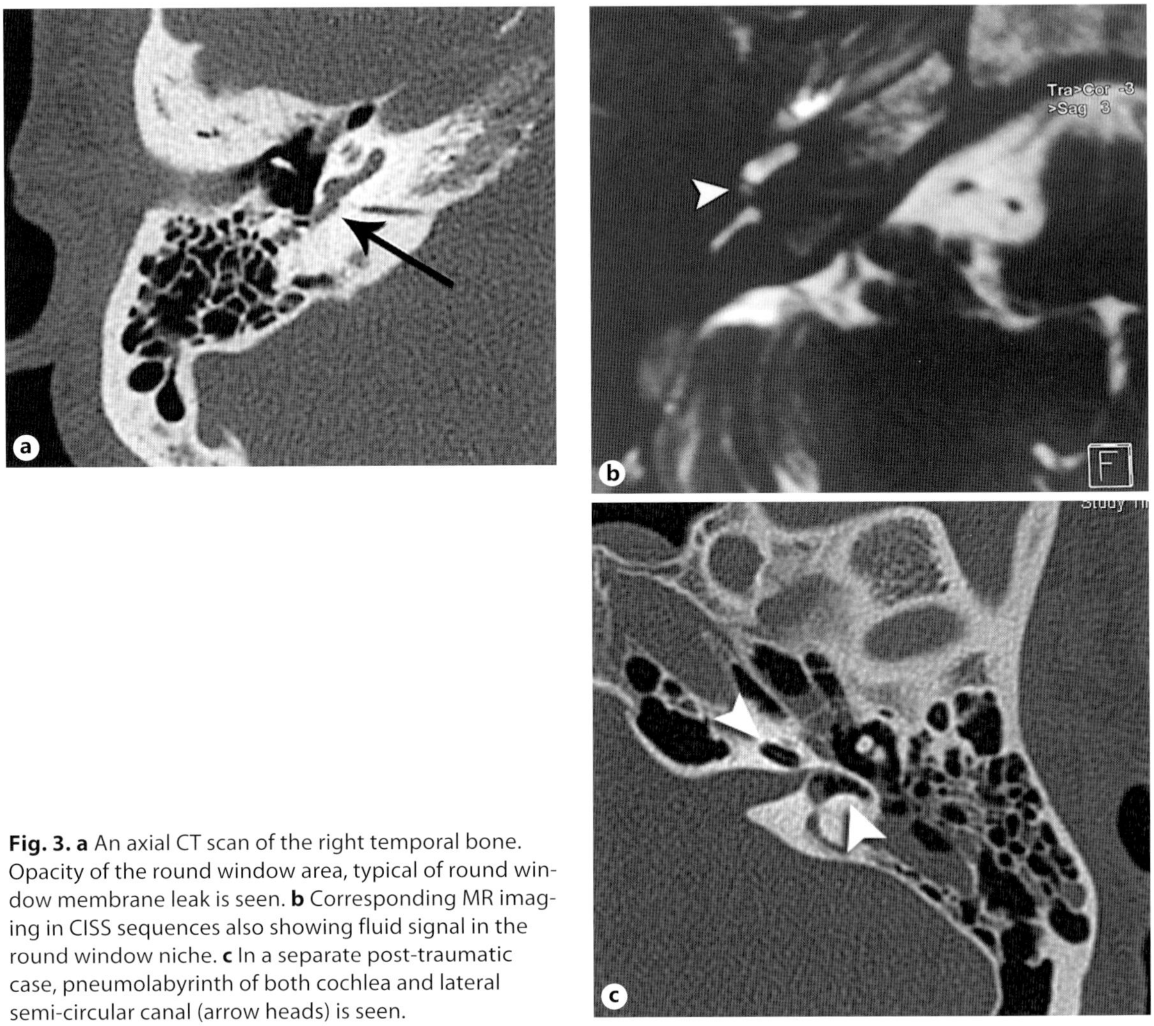

Fig. 3. a An axial CT scan of the right temporal bone. Opacity of the round window area, typical of round window membrane leak is seen. **b** Corresponding MR imaging in CISS sequences also showing fluid signal in the round window niche. **c** In a separate post-traumatic case, pneumolabyrinth of both cochlea and lateral semi-circular canal (arrow heads) is seen.

To improve the diagnosis rate, Benichou [24] used a variation of the threshold of the CT-scan gradient to identify PLF. In the same vein, King et al. [25] demonstrated the patency of the inner ear that occurred in 90% at the stapes area using MRI-scan with intra-tympanic administration of gadolinium [25].

Post-urography is a very sensitive evaluation tool, but lacks specificity. Its use in PLF assessment was described as early as 1992 [26]. Postural testing can be used in conjunction with exposure to noise and pressure changes to distinguish less obvious fistula-related dizziness [27]. It may also reveal an over-reliance on visual cues (visual dependency) that reflect vestibular impairment (Fig. 4). We thus think that using post-urography along with wavelet analysis may help demonstrate both slight impairment of sway (Fig. 5), and malingering when facing periodic oscillation of the centre of gravity that can be revealed by the analysis in frequency domain.

All these investigations are useful but are time consuming. Thus, the decision to select one or more of these tests should be undertaken on a case-by-case basis, depending on the severity of symptoms, especially auditory. In cases with a

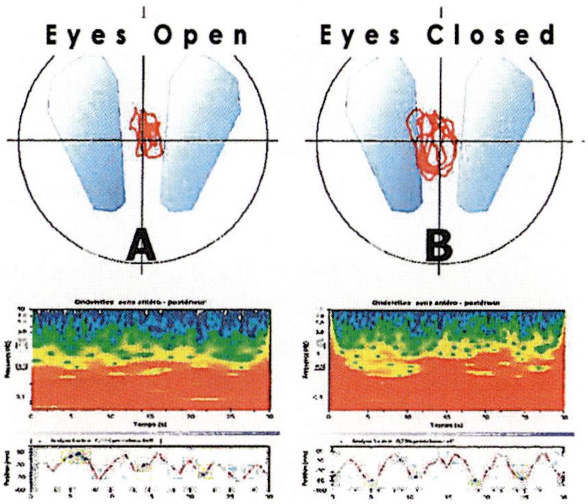

Fig. 4. Global results of the post-urography test. At the top, the relevant values for afferent outputs (somesthetic, visual and vestibular) are shown as well as the resultant dependency on visual cues (which, in a normal patient, should be minimal). At the bottom are charts demonstrating the corresponding values of the energy devoted to accomplish the tasks, across the frequency domain (wavelet analysis). The greater the energy (red), the lesser the capacity to maintain posture.

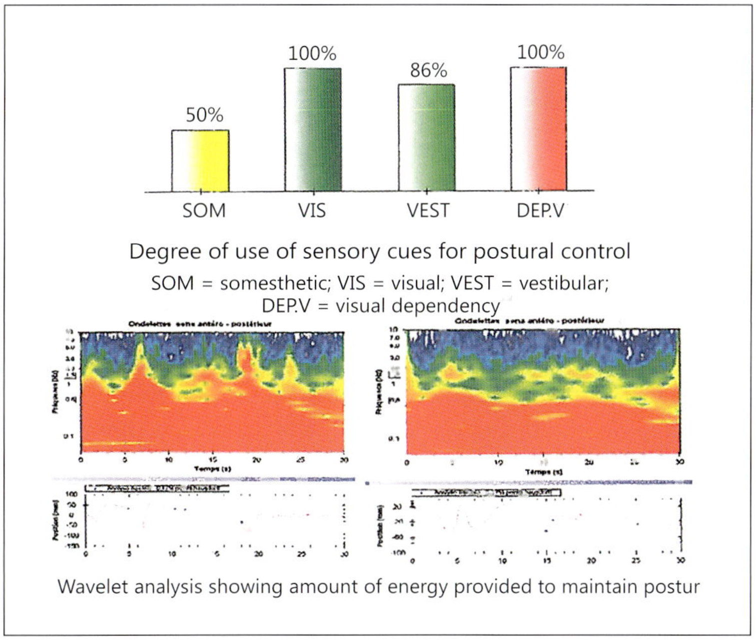

Fig. 5. Example of PLF revealed that a high energy is required to maintain posture even in the eyes open condition with a stable board. The difference in the energy domain is not significant when the eyes are closed, demonstrating significant impairment of the vestibular control.

clear clinical suspicion of PLF associated with a rapidly progressive decrease in hearing thresholds, surgical exploration should not be delayed.

The gold standard means of making a diagnosis is direct visualization of the perilymphatic leak through a tympanotomy. This is, often both difficult and highly subjective (see below).

A Novel Biomarker CTP for PLF Diagnosis, Japanese Diagnostic Criteria and Nationwide Survey

A number of markers have been used to aid diagnosis of PLF. This includes beta-2 transferrin, beta-trace protein (prostaglandin D synthase)

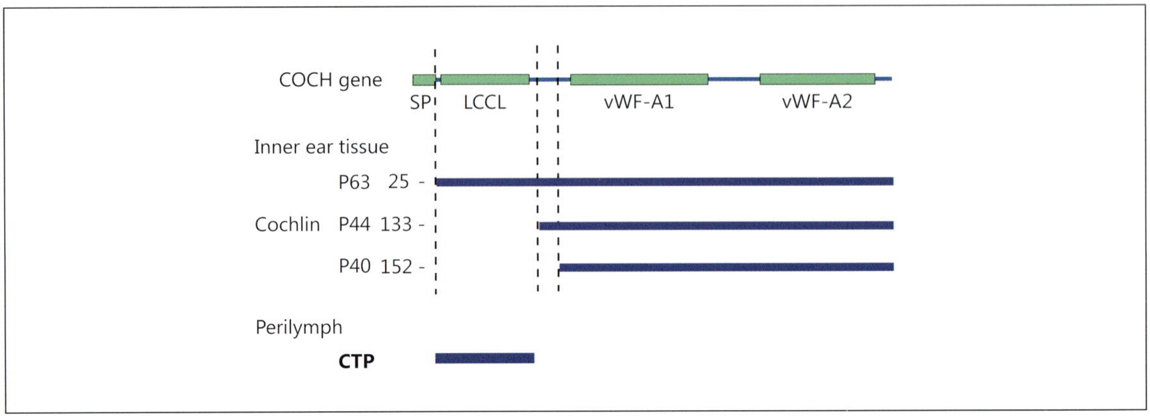

Fig. 6. Illustrated primary molecular structure of Cochlin isoforms in inner ear and perilymph (modified from ref. [13]; Fig. 1a). Representation of the COCH gene and Cochlin protein. The top line denotes the deduced amino acid sequence of human COCH, showing the positions of the signal peptide (SP), the limulus factor C, Cochlin and the late gestation lung protein Lgl1 domain (LCCL), the intervening domains 1 and 2 (ivd1, 2), and the von Willebrand factor type A like domains 1 and 2 (vWF-A1, vWF-A2). The middle lines depict bovine Cochlin isoforms, p63s, p44s and p40s, expressed in inner ear tissue. The numbers of the N-terminal amino acid of each isoform are indicated. The bottom line depicts the Cochlin-tomoprotein (CTP) isoform expressed in the perilymph.

and intrathecal fluorescein, all of which are markers of CSF leakage. An electrophoretic assay of middle ear fluid for the presence of beta-2 transferrin has been developed [28]. But whilst this technique holds promise, the dilutional effect during collection and preparation of the sample may lower the beta-2 transferrin concentration below the detection limits of the assay. Due to the relative amount of serum and perilymph in a mixed sample, electrophoretic separation of transferrin variant may not be diagnostic [29]. Similarly, beta-trace protein (Beta-TP, prostaglandin D synthase) has been used as a CSF leakage marker [30]. Beta-TP is detectable in higher concentrations in the inner ear fluids than in CSF. However, there are some difficulties with its use as the normal perilymph concentration of Beta-TP is unknown, and it is impossible to distinguish CSF leakage from PLF leakage [31, 32].

CTP is present in perilymph but not expressed in the serum, saliva or CSF. It has, therefore, been used as a novel biomarker for PLF [15] (Fig. 6). Leaked perilymph can be recovered by lavage of the middle ear with saline (MEL). The recovered fluid should preferably be more than 0.1 mL to allow for duplicate or triplicate measurements or re-testing, although 0.05 mL is the minimum volume that can be tested. In outpatients, MEL is collected after myringotomy using a conventional blade or CO2 laser. MEL can also be collected during surgery, such as exploratory tympanotomy, tympanoplasty or stapes surgery. When CTP is found in a sample, perilymph leakage is considered to be present. A negative test does not exclude a leak; however, it may indicate only a small volume of leakage or intermittent leakage.

Since 2009, Ikezono et al. [33, 34] have been using a western blot technique to test for CTP and have reported CTP in the cochlear fluid from patients with perilymph gushers via cochleostomy, from middle ear fluids following penetrating middle ear injuries and following revision stapes surgery [33–35]. In 2012, an ELISA kit using polyclonal antibodies was developed in collabo-

Table 2. Proposed Japanese diagnostic criteria of PLF (2017)

A	Symptoms Hearing impairment, tinnitus, aural fullness, vestibular symptoms are observed in those with the preceding events: (1) Coexisting or pre-existing middle and/or inner ear diseases, (trauma, cholesteatoma, tumor, anomaly, SCCD, etc.), middle and/or inner ear surgeries (2) Barotrauma caused by antecedent events of external origin (e.g., blasting, diving or flying, etc.) (3) Barotrauma caused by antecedent events of internal origin (e.g., nose-blowing, sneezing, straining or carrying heavy objects, etc)
B	Laboratory findings (1) Microscopic/Endoscopic inspection Visual identification of fistula(s) between middle and inner ear by microscope or endoscope. Fistulas can develop at the cochlear window, vestibular window, fracture site; microfissure, malformation, destruction in bony labyrinth caused by inflammation, etc. (2) Biochemical test Perilymph-specific protein is detected from the middle ear
C	Reference (1) A perilymph specific protein; e.g., Cochlin-tomoprotein (CTP) detection test. After myringotomy, the middle ear is rinsed with 0.3 ml saline 3 times; the fluid is recovered (middle ear lavage (MEL)) and tested by polyclonal antibody ELISA. The cut-off criteria: $\sim 0.4 < \text{CTP}$ negative; $0.4 \leqq \text{CTP} < 0.8$ intermediate; $0.8 \leqq \text{CTP}$ positive (2) Idiopathic cases may exist. (3) Following symptoms and/or test results may be observed: 1 Streaming water-like tinnitus or feeling of running water in the middle ear 2 Popping sound can be heard at the onset 3 Nystagmus and/or vertigo induced by pressure application to the middle ear (Hennebert's phenomenon, fistula sign) 4 Imaging studies may show a fistula in the bony labyrinth or pneumolabyrinth 5 Progression of hearing impairment, tinnitus, aural fullness may be acute, progressive, fluctuating or recurrent 6 The main complaints can be vestibular symptoms without hearing impairment
D	Differential diagnosis Inner ear diseases with known causes, such as viral infection, genetic, vestibular schwannoma, etc.
E	Diagnosis Probable PLF: Only symptoms listed in A Definite PLF: Symptoms and laboratory findings listed in B

ration with IBL (Immuno-Biological Laboratories, Inc., Gunma, Japan). This has been used to test samples from 100 hospitals nationwide with the help of SRL, Inc., one of the biggest clinical laboratory testing service enterprises in Japan. This technique is more straightforward than the previously described western blot testing system, with results easily reported to the patient's clinician [36, 37].

Unlike other countries, PLF has been one of the main targets for otology research in Japan. The first diagnostic criteria was put forward in 1983 [38] and since then, a national study group has been studying PLF. After the introduction of the diagnostic test using CTP, PLF diagnostic criteria were revised in 2016 [37] (Table 2). It is based on clinical symptoms, history and physiological test results. Figure 7 shows the ratio of cas-

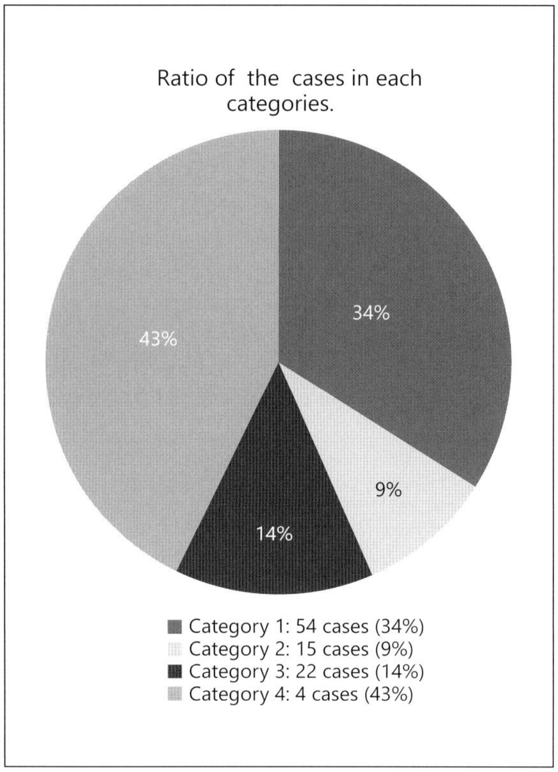

Fig. 7. The ratio of categories of diagnosis in cases.

es by diagnostic category in the recent national study. The high proportion of category 4 patients (idiopathic) reflects the fact that Japanese ENT physicians are accustomed to suspecting PLF. Seven to 20% of the cases in each category showed CTP positive test results. These results clearly indicate that PLF is a real clinical entity.

What Therapeutic Strategy Could be Proposed?

Although surgical intervention is the key treatment option, it is not always necessary. Close follow-up of patients can be recommended along with preventive measures (avoiding elevation of inner ear pressure and cranial pressure) when there is minimal impact on the quality of life and normal or stable hearing. Such an attitude is justified by the fact that there may be spontaneous resolution of symptoms. Before progressing to surgical sealing, intra-tympanic steroid administration may be considered. This can be effective in acute decompensation of Meniere's disease, labyrinthitis and PLF. It is important to consider that the effectiveness of trans-tympanic therapy may be limited if sealing of the labyrinthine windows is undertaken.

It is important to realize that although several potential pathways exist between the perilymphatic space and the middle ear, the actual leakage of fluid can be difficult or impossible to prove [39]. The conventional gold standard of PLF detection is the intraoperative visualization of perilymph leakage. This is not always possible, however, and the absence of observed leakage does not exclude the diagnosis. Similarly, the presence of fluid collection in the round and oval window niches may not necessarily represent perilymph as blood, tissue fluid and irrigation fluid can all be mistaken for perilymph [40]. The difficulty of making a definitive diagnosis of PLF has caused a long-standing debate regarding its prevalence, natural history, management and even its very existence [1, 2, 41–43].

Surgical Technique

In the presence of disabling symptoms (vertigo and dizziness, progressive sensorineural hearing loss), surgical sealing of the fistula is recommended. This is achieved through middle ear exploration, ideally using both microscope and endoscope. Leakage from the oval and round window areas is sought and systematic sealing of the windows undertaken even if no leakage is identified. Autologous connective tissue is harvested and used to obliterate oval and round windows. Fat, temporalis fascia or perichondrium from the tragus can all be used. The latter is our material of choice considering its ease of use and relative sta-

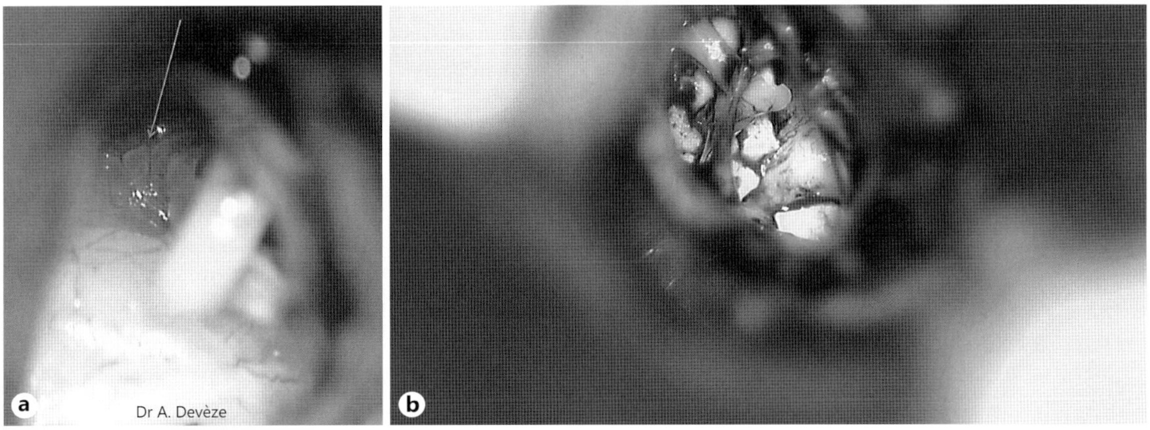

Fig. 8. a Example of a malformation of the left footplate area. A breach (arrow) is seen at the anterior part of the footplate (**b**). Intraoperative picture of a right ear. After elevation of the drum, sealing of both oval and round window areas was carried out using perichondrium after refreshing surrounding mucosa.

bility in fluids (fascia has the disadvantage that it swells in contact with fluid). Counseling of the patient is crucial and patients should be informed that a specific leak may not be identified, but that sealing will be undertaken even if this is the case. Hyperventilation, Trendeleberg positioning and jugular vein compression can be used to increase diagnostic yield but are not necessarily effective (Fig. 8).

Prognosis appears to be linked to the delay between the causative event and surgical treatment [44]; however, it seems difficult to reduce this delay to intervention. Despite this, some patients may benefit from surgical treatment up to 6 months after the causative event [45, 46].

Conclusion

To conclude, PLF is a genuine condition that requires a high index of suspicion to identify cases. Every case of suspected PLF requires a thorough evaluation through clinical assessment and investigation. The work-up should ideally include audiovestibular investigations with positional audiometry, videonystagmography with Tullio and Valsalva testing and cVEMP as a minimum. Cross-sectional imaging should also be undertaken. The CTP test is currently being reviewed for Japanese FDA approval, and may become available worldwide in several years as a useful adjunct to diagnosis. Close communication between radiologist, clinicians, surgeons and the patient is crucial and represents one of the key points of this particular disease.

Acknowledgments

We thank Ms. Miki Hatakeyama for editorial assistance with the production of this manuscript.

Source of Funding

This study was supported by Health and Labor Sciences Research Grants in Japan (Research on Measures for Intractable Diseases, Researches on Sensory and Communicative Disorders).

References

1 Hornibrook J: Perilymph fistula: fifty years of controversy. ISRN Otolaryngol 2012;2012:281248.

2 Schuknecht HF: Myths in neurotology. Am J Otol 1992;13:124–126.

3 Meyerhoff WL: Spontaneous perilymphatic fistula: myth or fact. Am J Otol 1993;14:478–481.

4 Jackler R, Brackmann D: Neurotology, ed 2. Philadelphia, Pennsylvania, Mosby Inc., 2005.

5 Minor LB: Labyrinthine fistulae: pathobiology and management. Curr Opin Otolaryngol Head Neck Surg 2003;11: 340–346.

6 Maitland CG: Perilymphatic fistula. Curr Neurol Neurosci Rep 2001;1:486–491.

7 Wackym P, Balaban C, Mackay H, Wood S, Lundell C, Carter D, et al: Longitudinal cognitive and neurobehavioral functional outcomes before and after repairing otic capsule dehiscence. Otol Neurotol 2016;37:70–82.

8 Bourgeois B, Ferron Ch, Bordure P, Beauvillain de Montreuil C, Legent F: [Exploratory tympanotomy for suspected traumatic perilymphatic fistula]. Ann Otolaryngol Chir Cervicofac 2005;122: 181–186.

9 Goto F, Ogawa K, Kunihiro T, Kurashima K, Kobayashi H, Kanzaki J: Perilymph fistula – 45 case analysis. Auris Nasus Larynx 2001;28:29–33.

10 Fitzgerald DC: Perilymphatic fistula and Meniere's disease. Clinical series and literature review. Ann Otol Rhinol Laryngol 2001;110(5 pt 1):430–436.

11 Stroud MH, Calcaterra TC: Spontaneous perilymph fistulas. Laryngoscope 1970; 80:479–487.

12 Portmann D, Souza Leao F, Bussieres R, Noyon P: [Validation of a clinical scale for the diagnosis of perilymphatic fistula]. Rev Laryngol Otol Rhinol (Bord) 2005;126:243–248.

13 Ikezono T, Shindo S, Li L, Omori A, Ichinose S, Watanabe A, et al: Identification of a novel Cochlin isoform in the perilymph: insights to Cochlin function and the pathogenesis of DFNA9. Biochem Biophys Res Commun 2004;314:440–446.

14 Ikezono T, Shindo S, Sekiguchi S, Hanprasertpong C, Li L, Pawankar R, et al: Cochlin-tomoprotein: a novel perilymph-specific protein and a potential marker for the diagnosis of perilymphatic fistula. Audiol Neurotol 2009;14: 338–344.

15 Ikezono T, Shindo S, Sekiguchi S, Morizane T, Pawankar R, Watanabe A, et al: The performance of Cochlin-tomoprotein detection test for the diagnosis of perilymphatic fistula. Audiol Neurootol 2010;15:168–174.

16 Hazell JW, Fraser JG, Robinson PJ: Positional audiometry in the diagnosis of perilymphatic fistula. Am J Otol 1992; 13:263–269.

17 Albera R, Canale A, Lacilla M, Cavalot AL, Ferrero V: Delayed vertigo after stapes surgery. Laryngoscope 2004;114: 860–862.

18 Eggers S, Zee D: Overview of Vestibular and Balance Disorders. Handbook of Clinical Neurophysiology. Vertigo and Imbalance: Clinical Neurophysiology of the Vestibular System. Science Direct, 2010, vol 9, pp 3–4.

19 Modugno GC, Magnani G, Brandolini C, Savastio G, Pirodda A: Could vestibular evoked myogenic potentials (VEMPs) also be useful in the diagnosis of perilymphatic fistula? Eur Arch Otorhinolaryngol 2006;263:552–555.

20 Arenberg IK, Ackley RS, Ferraro J, Muchnik C: ECoG results in perilymphatic fistula: clinical and experimental studies. Otolaryngol Head Neck Surg 1988;99:435–443.

21 Marsot-Dupuch K, Gayet-Delacroix M: [Imaging of the cochleo-vestibular system]. J Radiol 1999;80:351–362.

22 Achache M, Sanjuan Puchol M, Santini L, Lafont B, Cihanek M, Lavieille JP, et al: Late pneumolabyrinth after undiagnosed post-traumatic perilymphatic fistula. Case report illustrating the importance of systematic emergency management.. Eur Ann Otorhinolaryngol Head Neck Dis 2013;130:283–287.

23 Veillon F, Rock B, Cahen-Riehm S, Meriot P, Charpiot A, Baur P; Imagerie de l'oreille traumatique. Imagerie de l'oreille et de l'os temporal. Paris, Lavoisier, 2014, pp 619–725.

24 Benichou J: Temporal Bone Imaging. Berlin, Springer, 2015.

25 King EB SA, Eastwood HT, O'Leary SJ. Direct entry of gadolinium into the vestibule following intratympanic applications in guinea pigs and the influence of cochlear implantation. J Assoc Res Otolaryngol 2011;12:741–751.

26 Shepard NT, Telian SA, Niparko JK, Kemink JL, Fujita S: Platform pressure test in identification of perilymphatic fistula. Am J Otol 1992;13:49–54.

27 Pyykkö I, Selmani Z, Zou J: Low-frequency sound pressure and transtympanic endoscopy of the middle ear in assessment of "spontaneous" perilymphatic fistula. ISRN Otolaryngol 2012; 2012:137623.

28 Bassiouny M, Hirsch BE, Kelly RH, Kamerer DB, Cass SP: Beta 2 transferrin application in otology. Am J Otol 1992; 13:552–555.

29 Rauch SD: Transferrin microheterogeneity in human perilymph. Laryngoscope 2000;110:545–552.

30 Bachmann G, Petereit H, Djenabi U, Michel O: Predictive values of beta-trace protein (prostaglandin D synthase) by use of laser-nephelometry assay for the identification of cerebrospinal fluid. Neurosurgery 2002;50:571–576.

31 Michel O, Petereit H, Klemm E, Walther LE, Bachmann-Harildstad G: First clinical experience with beta-trace protein (prostaglandin D synthase) as a marker for perilymphatic fistula. J Laryngol Otol 2005;119:765–769.

32 Risch L, Lisec I, Jutzi M, Podvinec M, Landolt H, Huber AR: Rapid, accurate and non-invasive detection of cerebrospinal fluid leakage using combined determination of beta-trace protein in secretion and serum. Clin Chim Acta 2005;351:169–176.

33 Ikezono T, Sugizaki K, Shindo S, Sekiguchi S, Pawankar R, Baba S, et al: CTP (Cochlin-tomoprotein) detection in the profuse fluid leakage (gusher) from cochleostomy. Acta Otolaryngol 2010;130: 881–887.

34 Ikezono T, Shindo S, Sekine K, Shiiba K, Matsuda H, et al: Cochlin-tomoprotein (CTP) detection test identifies traumatic perilymphatic fistula due to penetrating middle ear injury. Acta Otolaryngol 2011;131:937–944.

35 Kataoka Y, Ikezono T, Fukushima K, Yuen K, Maeda Y, Sugaya A, et al: Cochlin-tomoprotein (CTP) detection test identified perilymph leakage preoperatively in revision stapes surgery. Auris Nasus Larynx 2013;40:422–424.
36 Ikezono T, Matsumura T, Matsuda H, Shikaze S, Saitoh S, Shindo S, et al: The diagnostic performance of a novel ELISA for human CTP (Cochlin-tomoprotein) to detect perilymph leakage. PLoS One 2018;13:e0191498.
37 Matsuda H, Sakamoto K, Matsumura T, Saito S, Shindo S, Fukushima K, et al: A nationwide multicenter study of the Cochlin tomo-protein detection test: clinical characteristics of perilymphatic fistula cases. Acta Otolaryngol 2017; 137(suppl 565):S53–S59.
38 Kanzaki J: Diagnostic criteria for acute profound deafness. Acta Otolaryngol Suppl 1994;514:7–8.
39 Kohut RI, Hinojosa R, Budetti JA: Perilymphatic fistula: a histopathologic study. Ann Otol Rhinol Laryngol 1986; 95(5 pt 1):466–471.
40 Nomura Y: Perilymph fistula: concept, diagnosis and management. Acta Otolaryngol Suppl 1994;514:52–54.
41 Jackler R, Luxford W, House W. Congenital malformations of the inner ear: a classification based on embryogenesis. Laryngoscope 1987;97(3 pt 2 suppl 40):2–14.
42 Friedland DR, Wackym PA: A critical appraisal of spontaneous perilymphatic fistulas of the inner ear. Am J Otol 1999; 20:261–276; discussion 276–279.
43 Hughes GB, Sismanis A, House JW: Is there consensus in perilymph fistula management? Otolaryngol Head Neck Surg 1990;102:111–117.
44 Kubo T, Kohno M, Naramura H, Itoh M: Clinical characteristics and hearing recovery in perilymphatic fistulas of different etiologies. Acta Otolaryngol (Stockh) 1993;113:307–311.
45 Glasscock ME 3rd, Hart MJ, Rosdeutscher JD, Bhansali SA: Traumatic perilymphatic fistula: how long can symptoms persist? A follow-up report. Am J Otol 1992;13:333–338.
46 Gedlicka C, Formanek M, Ehrenberger K: Analysis of 60 patients after tympanotomy and sealing of the round window membrane after acute unilateral sensorineural hearing loss. Am J Otolaryngol 2009;30:157–161.

Prof. Tetsuo Ikezono, MD, PhD
Saitama Medical University Faculty of Medicine, Otorhinolaryngology
Morohongo 38, Moroyamamachi
Irumagun, Saitamaken 350-0495 (Japan)
E-Mail ikez@saitama-med.ac.jp

What is ETD?

ETD is one of the most common problems seen in ENT clinics, with an estimated prevalence around 1% in adults [12]. The prevalence in children is probably higher. Ventilation tube insertion for persistent OME is one of the most common operations performed in children, but we still do not have a complete understanding of the importance of ETD in OME; although it is generally agreed that it is a contributory factor. Given the prevalence of ETD, it is surprising that, in general, the diagnosis of ETD has relied on clinical judgement rather than a set of defined criteria. Definition of ETD is challenging as there are different forms of ETD and the symptoms vary and are non-specific, being common to many different forms of middle and inner ear pathologies. These include aural fullness, popping or cracking, discomfort, hearing loss, tinnitus and autophony. The lack of criteria for diagnosis of ETD is also due to a poor understanding of the function of the Eustachian tube and the general lack of research in the field, in part due to the poor efficacy of interventions to treat ETD. The relatively recent invention of a potential treatment for ETD in the form of BET has led to renewed interest in the field.

The first international consensus on the definition, clinical presentation and diagnosis of ETD was recently published, reporting on a meeting of experts in the field that took place at a workshop in June 2014 [13]. It should be noted that this applies only to adults and, importantly, not to other middle ear diseases such as OME, chronic suppurative otitis media, tympanic membrane retraction and cholesteatoma. ETD was defined as symptoms and signs of pressure dysregulation in the middle ear, with chronic ETD diagnosed where these are present for at least three months. Acute dilatory (obstructive) ETD often follows an upper respiratory tract infection and is probably due to inflammation of the mucosa lining the Eustachian tube, which may become chronic. Baro-challenge induced ETD describes the same symptoms experienced with changes in pressure, commonly with flying or diving. Patulous ETD is characterized by autophony and symptoms may improve when lying down. The symptoms common to all forms of ETD are aural fullness, popping or pain. Signs include evidence of a negative middle ear pressure, either with tympanometry or otoscopic appearances of the tympanic membrane, such as retraction. However, this is further complicated as many patients have symptoms of ETD without signs of middle ear disease and standard tympanometry may be normal, particularly in patulous ETD. While tympanometry is a sensitive and specific measure of OME, there are limited data on the accuracy of tympanometry for ETD [14]. It remains to be seen whether this definition will become accepted by the wider international community.

How Do We Measure ETD?

There are many different tests of ETD and evidence for use of the majority is weak. There have been many attempts to develop objective tests for ETD [15], but no single test has been found to be a reliable diagnostic tool [16]. With the development of treatments such as BET that may more directly address the underlying cause of ETD by aiming to improve the function of the Eustachian tube, a better understanding of available tests for ETD and their sensitivity and specificity is required. A narrative systematic review of tests of ETD has recently been published and the results are summarized below [17]. It should be noted that the accuracy of tests reported is difficult to compare since ETD is defined differently in nearly every study.

The ideal test of ETD should be non-invasive and measure function over a prolonged period, as it has been shown that individual middle ear pressures can vary considerably within a relative time frame in both healthy individuals and those with ETD [18]. Otoscopy demonstrates the presence of chronic ear disease, but is an insensitive method of assessing the physiology of Eustachian tube opening. The majority of tests available to assess ETD involve assessing whether a change in pressure in either the nasopharynx or external ear canal result in opening of the Eustachian tube. The pressure change can be applied through the external ear canal, nose, by the patient through swallowing, or by maneuvers such a Valsalva (forced exhalation against a closed nose and mouth), Toynbee (swallow while nose occluded) or a sniff (rapid inhalation though the nose).

Tympanometry is the simplest and most widely available method used to assess ETD and uses the application of pressure in the external ear canal. As described previously, there are poor data on accuracy for measuring ETD, and a single measure of middle ear pressure is of limited value as this varies considerably over a few hours [19].

Where tympanometry is used to measure pressure changes after Valsalva, Toynbee or sniff, sensitivity for ETD is between 50 and 70% [20, 21].

A weakness of patient applied maneuvers is the variability in pressure applied by the patient. Tubo-tympan-aerodynamic-graphy assesses this by including a nasal probe to measure pressure in the nasopharynx when maneuvers are performed, as well as a probe to measure impedance in the ear. However, these tests still rely on passive opening of the Eustachian tube due to the pressure created in the nasopharynx, rather than active opening of the Eustachian tube through contraction of peritubal muscles when swallowing, which is more representative of normal physiological opening. Tubomanometry applies a standardized pressure to the nasopharynx through a nasal applicator. An active swallowing by the patient is performed at the same time as a defined pressure (usually 30, 40, or 50 mbar) is applied through the nose to the nasopharynx, with any resulting change in pressure detected in the ear canal. While this determines whether the Eustachian tube has opened, it is the latency from when the pressure is applied in the nasopharynx to when a rise in pressure is detected in the middle ear that appears to be most useful, with a sensitivity of 87% and specificity of 67% for identifying ETD [22].

The weakness of all the methods described is the application of an artificial pressure, whether by the patient or delivered externally to the ear or nasopharynx. Sonotubometry is an interesting method that measures the passage of sound through the Eustachian tube to determine whether it has opened when the patient swallows, a phenomenon first described by Politzer in 1865. A speaker delivers sound through the nares, which passes into the nasopharynx, through the Eustachian tube when it opens, into the middle ear and is detected by a microphone in the external ear canal. This allows the assessment of Eustachian tube opening under more normal physiological conditions. However, sensitivity for ETD remains low at 53%, although specificity is high at 91% [23]. In addition, sound transmission is not a normal function of the Eustachian tube and 10–20% of healthy individuals have no detectable opening during swallowing.

Radiological assessment of the Eustachian tube offers a non-invasive means of assessing ETD and a systematic review on this subject has recently been published [24]. While both CT and MRI can give some information on anatomical obstruction of the Eustachian tube or features suggestive of a patulous Eustachian tube, it is dynamic imaging that has the potential to assess function. However, current protocols have yet to demonstrate reliable information that is clinically useful and there is currently insufficient evidence to recommend imaging as part of a routine assessment of ETD.

Patient questionnaires offer an attractive method of assessing the symptoms that are seen in ETD. The ETDQ-7 was developed by assessing the differences between the answers to a set of questions between cases with ETD and controls [25]. High sensitivity (91%) and specificity (95%) was seen using a German translation in a case control study that far outperforms any of the objective tests described [26]. However, it is yet to be prospectively applied in a range of middle ear disorders.

Given the lack of any single test to measure ETD, it is likely that a combination of tests will be required to improve the accuracy of diagnosis and assess outcomes. The Eustachian Tube Score combines tubomanometry, patient-reported Valsalva and Toynbee, tympanometry and objective Valsalva to give 96% sensitivity and specificity of detecting ETD [27]. Further validation of objective tests combined with patient-reported questionnaires will allow the development of a core set of outcome measures to be used in trials of treatments for ETD.

How Can We Treat ETD

Medical Therapy

Currently, no medical therapies have shown efficacy in treating ETD [28]. The use of intranasal triamcinolone spray in patients with OME or negative middle ear pressure failed to show any difference compared to placebo controls in a randomized, double-blinded trial [29]. An earlier trial studied the effect of a decongestant agent versus placebo applied directly to the pharyngeal opening of the Eustachian tube, concluding that topical decongestant only improved Eustachian tube function at pressures higher than those normally encountered [30].

Surgery

Despite the widespread use of ventilation tubes (grommets) to treat ETD, there are no studies published evaluating their efficacy [28].

Laser tuboplasty of the Eustachian tube aims to remove the obstruction at the nasopharyngeal entrance of the Eustachian tube. As such, it is only suitable for patients where hyperplasia of soft tissue is present at the ostium of the Eustachian tube, with otherwise normal function. This is performed endoscopically and can be carried out under local anesthesia in the outpatient setting. Otitis media with effusion was eliminated in 40% of adults at two years when combined with medical therapy [29].

BET is a minimally invasive method that aims to treat chronic obstructive ETD by dilating the Eustachian tube with a balloon under general anesthesia. The balloon catheter is introduced into the Eustachian tube via the nose, under transnasal endoscopic vision. Once the balloon is correctly positioned in the cartilaginous portion of the Eustachian tube, it is filled with saline up to a pressure of 10 bars for 2 min and then deflated and removed (Fig. 1).

There is a growing body of experience in this field with over 20,000 procedures performed worldwide. No significant complications have been reported, with 3 cases of subcutaneous emphysema in 622 cases of BET in the largest series published to date [30]. Carotid injury is the main potential complication of concern in BET. However, this has not been reported, and the balloons should only sit in the cartilaginous portion of the Eustachian tube. In terms of efficacy, BET has shown improvement in 70–80% of patients at 1 year [30–32]. However, these case series had mixed indications and inclusion criteria, no control groups and mixed outcome measures. Currently, there is insufficient evidence to make firm conclusions regarding the efficacy of BET for treating specific indications, such as OME or retraction pockets. Although BET is a promising treatment for ETD, studies are hampered by a lack of robust outcome measures. The development of a core set of outcome measures for ETD is required to facilitate trials in the future [17].

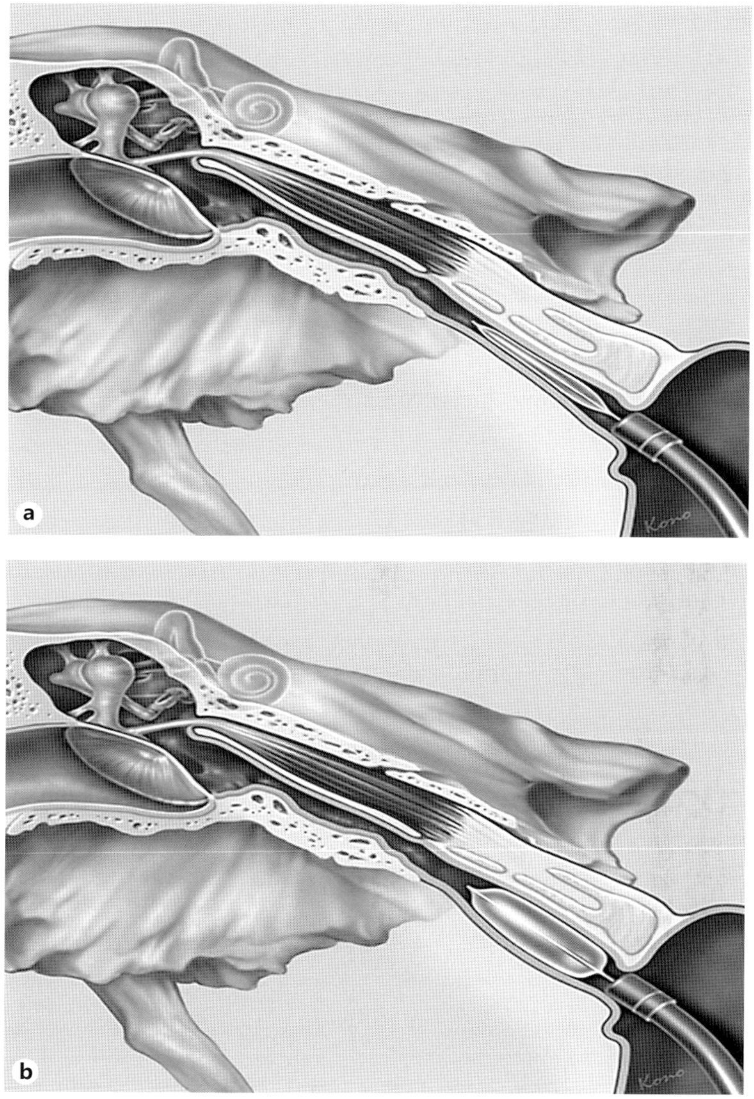

Fig. 1. a, b Balloon Eustachian tuboplasty.

Conclusions

The Eustachian tube is an important factor in the development of middle ear disease. However, its role in different forms of middle ear pathology is currently not understood. To further the field, we need a definition of ETD and robust outcome methods to perform and compare trials of promising treatments, such as BET. A recent international consensus has published a definition and many groups, including ours, are working towards a better understanding of the measurement of ETD. BET represents the most promising treatment for ETD and has a good safety profile. The results of controlled trials will allow us to determine the efficacy of BET in treating middle ear disease in the near future.

References

1 Prades JM, et al: Descriptive anatomy of the human auditory tube. Surg Radiol Anat 1998;20:335–340.

2 Robert Y, Gaillandre L, Chaillet N, Francke JP: [Anatomy of the auditory tube: CT scan and MRI aspect]. Ann Radiol (Paris) 1992;35:444–452.

3 Takasaki K, et al: Measurement of angle and length of the Eustachian tube on computed tomography using the multiplanar reconstruction technique. Laryngoscope 2007;117:1251–1254.

4 Poe DS, Pyykkö I, Valtonen H, Silvola J: Analysis of Eustachian tube function by video endoscopy. Am J Otol 2000;21: 602–607.

5 Alper CM, Swarts JD, Singla A, Banks J, Doyle WJ: Relationship between the electromyographic activity of the paratubal muscles and Eustachian tube opening assessed by sonotubometry and videoendoscopy. Arch Otolaryngol Head Neck Surg 2012;138:741–746.

6 Sudo M, Sando I, Suzuki C: Three-dimensional reconstruction and measurement study of human Eustachian tube structures: a hypothesis of Eustachian tube function. Ann Otol Rhinol Laryngol 1998;107:547–554.

7 CD B: Eustachian Tube Structure, Function, Role in Otitis Media. Lewiston, NY, BC Decker, 2005.

8 Licameli GR: The Eustachian tube. Update on anatomy, development, and function. Otolaryngol Clin North Am 2002;35:803–809.

9 Amoodi H, Bance M, Thamboo A: Magnetic resonance imaging illustrating change in the Ostmann fat pad with age. J Otolaryngol Head Neck Surg 2010;39: 440–441.

10 Sadé J, Ar A: Middle ear and auditory tube: middle ear clearance, gas exchange, and pressure regulation. Otolaryngol Head Neck Surg 1997;116:499–524.

11 Mondain M, Vidal D, Bouhanna S, Uziel A: Monitoring Eustachian tube opening: preliminary results in normal subjects. Laryngoscope 1997;107:1414–1419.

12 Browning GG, Gatehouse S: The prevalence of middle ear disease in the adult British population. Clin Otolaryngol Allied Sci 1992;17:317–321.

13 Schilder AGM, et al: Eustachian tube dysfunction: consensus statement on definition, types, clinical presentation and diagnosis. Clin Otolaryngol 2015;40: 407–411.

14 Bluestone CD, Beery QC, Paradise JL: Audiometry and tympanometry in relation to middle ear effusions in children. Laryngoscope 1973;83:594–604.

15 Holmquist J, Olén L: Evaluation of Eustachian tube function. J Laryngol Otol 1980;94:15–23.

16 Llewellyn A, et al: Interventions for adult Eustachian tube dysfunction: a systematic review. Health Technol Assess 2014;18:1–180, v–vi.

17 Smith ME, Tysome JR: Tests of Eustachian tube function: a review. Clin Otolaryngol 2015;40:300–311.

18 Grøntved A, et al: Monitoring middle ear pressure by tympanometry. A study of middle ear pressure variation through seven hours. Acta Otolaryngol 1989;108: 101–106.

19 Falk B: Negative middle ear pressure induced by sniffing. A tympanometric study in persons with healthy ears. J Otolaryngol 1981;10:299–305.

20 Kumazawa T, et al: Eustachian tube function tests and their diagnostic potential in normal and diseased ears. Acta Otolaryngol Suppl 1993;500:10–13.

21 Kumazawa T, Honjo I, Honda K: Aerodynamic pattern of Eustachian tube dysfunction. Arch Otorhinolaryngol 1977; 215,317–323.

22 Esteve D: Tubomanometry and pathology; in Ars B (ed): Fibrocartilaginous Eustachian Tube: Middle Ear Cleft. The Hague, Netherlands, Kugler Publications, 2003, pp 159–175.

23 Asenov DR, et al: Sonotubometry with perfect sequences: first results in pathological ears. Acta Otolaryngol 2010;130: 1242–1248.

24 Smith ME, Scoffings DJ, Tysome JR: Imaging of the Eustachian tube and its function: a systematic review. Neuroradiology 2016;58:543–556.

25 McCoul ED, Anand VK, Christos PJ: Validating the clinical assessment of Eustachian tube dysfunction: The Eustachian Tube Dysfunction Questionnaire (ETDQ-7). Laryngoscope 2012;122: 1137–1141.

26 Schröder S, Lehmann M, Sudhoff H, Ebmeyer J: [Assessment of chronic obstructive Eustachian tube dysfunction: evaluation of the German version of the Eustachian Tube Dysfunction Questionnaire]. HNO 2014;62:160, 162–164.

27 Schröder S, Lehmann M, Sauzet O, Ebmeyer J, Sudhoff H: A novel diagnostic tool for chronic obstructive Eustachian tube dysfunction – the Eustachian tube score. Laryngoscope 2015;125:703–708.

28 Norman G, et al: Systematic review of the limited evidence base for treatments of Eustachian tube dysfunction: a health technology assessment. Clin Otolaryngol 2014;39:6–21.

29 Poe DS, Grimmer JF, Metson R: Laser Eustachian tuboplasty: two-year results. Laryngoscope 2007;117:231–237.

30 Schröder S, Lehmann M, Ebmeyer J, Upile T, Sudhoff H: Balloon Eustachian tuboplasty: a retrospective cohort study. Clin Otolaryngol 2015;40:629–638.

31 Dalchow CV, et al: First results of Endonasal dilatation of the Eustachian tube (EET) in patients with chronic obstructive tube dysfunction. Eur Arch Otorhinolaryngol 2016;273:607–613.

32 Tisch M, Maier S, Maier H: [Eustachian tube dilation using the Bielefeld balloon catheter: clinical experience with 320 interventions]. HNO 2013;61:483–487.

James R. Tysome
ENT Department, Box 48, Addenbrooke's Hospital
Hills Road
Cambridge CB2 0QQ (UK)
E-Mail jrt20@cam.ac.uk

Author Index

Subject Index